J. Lawrence Driskill

Adventures in Senior Living
Learning How to Make Retirement Meaningful and Enjoyable

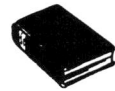

*Pre-publication
REVIEWS,
COMMENTARIES,
EVALUATIONS . . .*

"Larry Driskill has done it again! Weaving together interviews of retirees in 'their own words,' he has demonstrated his skill as a good listener and a storyteller par excellence.

In contrast to the literature produced by business and government agencies, retirement is presented as a hopeful and joyful adventure. Rather than having time hanging heavily on their hands, these retirees lend a hand by volunteering their much-needed experience and caring.

Not without elements of sadness, their true-to-life experiences are testimonies to God's faithfulness as well as the perseverance of the saints. For me, the main gift of this book is not allowing their stories to go untold."

Pasquale A. Castellano, DMin
Pastor, Calvary Presbyterian Church, South Pasadena, CA

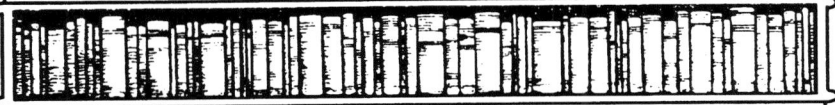

More pre-publication
REVIEWS, COMMENTARIES, EVALUATIONS . . .

"This is an upbeat book, fulfilling well its purpose to be helpful to persons in or facing retirement. The content consists of interviews conducted by Dr. Driskill with thirty-one persons, all with experience in retirement. A majority are residents of Westminster Gardens (as is Dr. Driskill), a retirement home operated by the Presbyterian Church (U.S.A.). Almost all are persons with long years of professional service in the church, especially as overseas missionaries. They represent high levels of spiritual as well as educational and cultural maturity. In one sense the book is from an elite group aiming to help others achieve happy lifestyles that are also helpful to others.

This book, however, is eminently practical, replete with advice, especially focusing on volunteer service to others. In spite of the high spiritual and cultural background of those interviewed, there is really no condescension in their sharing of experiences past and present. Not a few retirees stressed the importance of cultivating personal relationships with spouses, friends, neighbors, and above all with God. The book is not pious in tone, but almost all retirees 'indicate that faith in God helps them in facing aging and retirement problems . . . faith that God will guide and help them through difficult times.'

To the above may be added the observation that continuing education seems to be a goal for many retirees. Much is said of the importance of recreation and exercise—very little on diet! The importance of a sense of humor is stressed, by both retirees and the interviewer. All in all, the book is highly recommended, even for all ages."

Richard Henry Drummond, PhD
Professor of Ecumenical Mission and History of Religions, Emeritus, University of Dubuque Theological Seminary, Dubuque, IA

"By describing the flesh and blood of real seniors' experiences, Larry Driskill has made it possible to discern the underlying skeletal structure that gives stability and balance to retirement years. This structure includes planning, cultivating interests and friends, volunteerism that brings fulfillment, a new calling for caregivers of spouses, and continual mental and spiritual growth. Because the people are real, the readers can find a wealth of practical models to enhance their maturing years."

J. Dudley Woodberry
Dean, School of World Mission, Fuller Theological Seminary, Pasadena, CA

More pre-publication
REVIEWS, COMMENTARIES, EVALUATIONS . . .

"**H**ave you ever wondered just what you would do in retirement? Larry Driskill's superbly crafted book of interviews of seniors in retirement is something every retired person will want to read. Larry has interviewed people with well-known names such as Christy Wilson, Jr., and ordinary people such as Dot Horcher or Ted Tajima. This book is full of great ideas for recreation (travel, reading, hiking); extending one's profession (teaching, evangelizing, ministering to needy folk); serving others (in their own home, hospitals, libraries, schools); and volunteering (providing food, clothing, and shelter, or even rehabilitation of prostitutes). One man spent one day a month taking different elderly people to lunch simply to give them a chance to be refreshed.

Larry has highlighted the fact that being busy is not the challenge for seniors; rather it is being active—in the service of others—that is the ultimate in self-enrichment. No senior needs to be bored during retirement and this book shows clearly just why that is true."

Marvin K. Mayers, PhD
Adjunct Professor of Anthropology,
Florida Gulf Coast University,
Southwest Florida

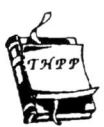

The Haworth Pastoral Press
An Imprint of The Haworth Press, Inc.

NOTES FOR PROFESSIONAL LIBRARIANS AND LIBRARY USERS

This is an original book title published by The Haworth Pastoral Press, an imprint of The Haworth Press, Inc. Unless otherwise noted in specific chapters with attribution, materials in this book have not been previously published elsewhere in any format or language.

CONSERVATION AND PRESERVATION NOTES

All books published by The Haworth Press, Inc. and its imprints are printed on certified ph neutral, acid free book grade paper. This paper meets the minimum requirements of American National Standard for Information Sciences–Permanence of Paper for Printed Material, ANSI Z39.48-1984.

Adventures in Senior Living
Learning How to Make Retirement Meaningful and Enjoyable

THE HAWORTH PASTORAL PRESS
Religion and Mental Health
Harold G. Koenig, MD
Senior Editor

New, Recent, and Forthcoming Titles:

Dying, Grieving, Faith, and Family: A Pastoral Care Approach **by George W. Bowman**

The Pastoral Care of Depression: A Guidebook **by Binford W. Gilbert**

Adventures in Senior Living: Learning How to Make Retirement Meaningful and Enjoyable **by J. Lawrence Driskill**

Adventures in Senior Living
Learning How to Make Retirement Meaningful and Enjoyable

Reverend J. Lawrence Driskill

The Haworth Pastoral Press
An Imprint of The Haworth Press, Inc.
New York • London

Published by

The Haworth Pastoral Press, an imprint of The Haworth Press, Inc., 10 Alice Street, Binghamton, NY 13904-1580

© 1997 by The Haworth Press, Inc. All rights reserved. No part of this work may be reproduced or utilized in any form or by any means, electronic or mechanical, including photocopying, microfilm, and recording, or by any information storage and retrieval system, without permission in writing from the publisher. Printed in the United States of America.

Cover design by Marylouise E. Doyle.

Library of Congress Cataloging-in-Publication Data

Driskill, J. Lawrence, 1920-
    Adventures in senior living : learning how to make retirement meaningful and enjoyable / J. Lawrence Driskill.
      p. cm
    Includes index.
    ISBN 0-7890-0253-1 (alk. paper).
      1. Aged volunteers—United States. 2. Aged volunteers—United States—Case studies. 3. Voluntarism—United States. 4. Voluntarism—Religious aspects—Christianity. 5. Retirement—United States. I. Title.
HV90.V64D74 1997
361.3′7′0846—dc21

                                                                     97-18763
                                                                      CIP

Gratefully dedicated
to those whose stories
appear in this book.

ABOUT THE AUTHOR

The Reverend J. Lawrence Driskill, STD, is a Pastor at the First Presbyterian Church, a Japanese-American church, of Altadena, California, where he provides services to the Japanese-speaking parishioners. He also performs voluntary work with other Asian-American churches in the Los Angeles area and is a Mission Advocate for San Gabriel Presbytery. Dr. Driskill first began working with Japanese people in the late 1940s while he was attending the San Francisco Theological Seminary in San Anselmo, California. In 1949, he was appointed by the former Board of Foreign Missions of the Presbyterian Church to carry on missionary work in the prefectural district of Osaka in Japan. His work there led to the establishment of several Christian groups, churches, Sunday schools, a nursery, a kindergarten, and Seikyo Gakuen Christian High School. Over the years, he has devoted much time and energy to teaching and strengthening the educational system at Seikyo Gakuen, as well as establishing new churches in a large housing complex north of Osaka City, where 170,100 white-collar workers live. Now age seventy-six, Dr. Driskill has written seven books in the last five years.

CONTENTS

Foreword	xi
Reverend Thomas C. Wentz	
Acknowledgments	xiii
Introduction	1
Nurse to African Babies, Then to American Retirees	3
Marabelle Taylor	
Caregiving for an Alzheimer's Spouse	7
Bob Lazear	
The Flower Lady	11
Eleanor Jamison	
Telephone Helpline and Shelter for Battered Women	15
Nannie Hereford	
The Library Lady	21
Mary Ruth Hoyt	
Recording Books on Tape for Blind People	27
Virginia Mackenzie	
A "Can't Say No" Volunteer	31
June Hansen	
A Retirement Ministry in Twenty-Five Countries	35
Paul Lindholm	
Helping Needy People and Prostitute Rescue Work	39
Faye Speer	
A Retirement Ministry Team	43
Hal and Kirby Davis	

Overcoming Grief While Helping Others   47
    Vicki McClelland Johnson

Pastoring, Writing, Singing, and Caring for Family   51
    Joe Gray

Retirement: Deceleration or Cold Turkey?   57
    Arthur Bushing

Planting a "Rose" in Westminster Gardens   61
    Bob McIntire and Gayle Beanland

Feeding and Caring for an Angel   65
    Henry (Tim) Lowe

Serving Navajos, Hawaiians, Alaskans,
and Yavapai-Apaches   69
    Jim Douthitt

Accomplishing a Musical "Dream" in Retirement   75
    Earle Harvey

Taking Widows and Widowers Out to Lunch   81
    Frank Jamison

Hospital Chaplain Work in Retirement   85
    Peter van Lierop

A Retired Teacher Who Didn't "Retire"   91
    Nelly Finch

Overcoming a Bad Beginning in Retirement   95
    Robert L. Caldwell

Retirement in Japan, Then in the United States   99
    Mildred (Millie) Brown

Choosing Variety in Work and in Retirement   105
    LeRoy (Roy) Engelhardt

Caring for God's Creation: Birds, Animals, and Humans *Helen Furgerson*	109
Helping Others and Overcoming Great Loss *Rhoda Iyoya*	115
Does a Housewife Retire? *Dot Horcher*	123
Surviving and Serving in Retirement *Ted Tajima*	131
Overcoming Internment and a Handicap, to Serve *Arthur Tsuneishi*	137
Helping to Evangelize People, Near and Far *Christy Wilson, Jr.*	143
Retirement: An Enjoyable Phase of Life *Bob and Peggy Thurman*	147
Sharing Stage and Screen Skills with Twentieth-Century Adventurers *Phyllis Love "Osanna" Gooding*	153
Insights Gained from These Retirees	161
Appendix: Graphs of Age Groups in the U.S.A. (from 1900 to 2030)	167
Glossary	171
Bibliography	173
Index	175

Foreword

A volunteer is one who imposes self-obligations.

Being a volunteer is what my parents called "doing the right thing." I remember being told by my parents to take a bag of groceries to a woman who lived back on the mountain behind our home in Hoagstown, Pennsylvania. It was cold and raining—and a long walk. I protested that I didn't know why we had to take responsibility for a woman I didn't even know. Why couldn't someone else do it? My mother's answer was that we knew of the need, and we would volunteer to meet it.

That is the way most of us have learned to volunteer, by example: seeing a need and meeting it. Volunteering individuals respond, not because it is required, but because the response is self-imposed.

In this country there is also a long tradition of organized voluntary service. It was the French historian Alexis de Tocqueville who commented so perceptively in *Democracy in America* on the peculiar American proclivity for organized volunteerism—not just individuals acts, but groups organized to perform volunteer service.

> These Americans are the most peculiar people in the world. You'll not believe it when I tell you how they behave. In a local community in their country, a citizen may conceive of some need which is not being met. What does he do? He goes across the street and discusses it with his neighbor. Then what happens? A committee comes into being and then the committee begins to function on behalf of the need. You won't believe this, but it's true; all of this is done by private citizens on their own initiative! (Conrad and Glenn, 1976, p. 2)

A distinctive mark of American society is the creation of voluntary associations. The notion of individuals who associate together for the common good is peculiarly, if not exclusively, an American tradition. Again it was De Tocqueville who observed the relationship between volunteerism and democracy: "The health of a democratic society may be measured by the quality of function performed by private citizens."

It is my observation, sharpened by more than thirty years of Christian ministry with those in retirement years, that those who are living in retirement are among the most active of volunteers. As demands for career and family lessen in middle life, opportunities for creative voluntary service increase.

Christians live with the biblical injunction to love one another. This is so whether they are in the first third of their life, when they are preparing for career and family; in the middle third, focused in vocation; or in the final third, retired.

At Westminster Gardens, a retirement community where I am currently the Executive Director, I have seen a unique coming together of the imperative for the Christian to love, the impulse of the American to volunteer, and the opportunity of the retired to live a lifestyle of voluntary obligation.

Westminster Gardens is a community comprised of those who have been professional providers of services. As a community, it is the finest example I have seen of people who continue to serve both individually and in organized groups. It is a community where obligations are self-imposed. Obligations are not placed by governmental regulation nor are they demanded through employment, but they are voluntarily—and happily—self-imposed.

This short book presents many life stories of extraordinary volunteerism, of service, of Christian impulse. I commend to you the reading of these illustrations of numerous acts of random kindness.

Reverend Thomas C. Wentz
Executive Director of Westminster Gardens

Acknowledgments

First, I want to thank those whose helpful retirement stories appear in this book. They are the ones who provided most of the information for this record of retirement adventures—good examples for all of us.

I also need to thank Ms. Osanna Love Gooding and the Westminster Gardens Writers' Group for their comments and suggestions. The Executive Director of Westminster Gardens, Reverend Thomas C. Wentz, kindly wrote the informative foreword, for which I am grateful.

Four Christian leaders provided helpful recommendations of the book to prospective readers: Dr. Thomas Gillespie, Dr. Clifton Kirkpatrick, Dr. Marsha Fowler, and Reverend Thomas C. Wentz.

And I am most grateful to my editor and publisher and to all those who helped make the publication of this book possible, especially Mrs. Betty Kiriyama, assisted by her husband George, who so kindly and skillfully put the book on a computer disk.

Most of all, I thank God who inspired the retirees presented here to "bear fruit in old age" (Psalm 92:14).

Introduction

Like death and taxes, retirement comes to all of us—if we live long enough. Now one in eight Americans is age sixty-five or over, according to a report on the *NBC Evening News*, May 20, 1996. For every sixty-five men there are one hundred women over age sixty-five. In an earlier NBC report I learned that about half of all retired people do some volunteer work. But that means that the other half does not do volunteer work—some because they cannot and others for various reasons. The retirement stories in this book illustrate, however, how important volunteer work is—for those who receive help and those who give it. Quite clearly, everyone benefits. As indicated in the appendix of this book, senior citizens are the fastest growing segment of American society. Therefore, we not only need to provide for their needs but we also benefit from their increasingly important contribution to our society.

In her retirement story, Mary Ruth Hoyt reminds us how our retirement can be much more meaningful and enjoyable if we plan ahead for it—especially with good economic planning. In his story, Peter van Lierop tells us that while our main retirement activities should center around areas in which we have training and experience, we should not be afraid to try new things.

Bob Lazear gives his example of a retiree who must devote most retirement time to caring for a sick spouse, relative, or friend. Bob says, "God has given me a new 'calling' in retirement: The full-time vocation of caring for my Alzheimer's wife—dressing her in the morning, watching and feeding her all day, and putting her to bed at night."

As health costs skyrocket, many of us may have to care for ill people at home. But we can also, as Eleanor Jamison reminds us, brighten the lives of patients in nursing homes or hospitals as much-needed volunteers. In that volunteer service, we can find our own retirement life enriched.

I know, and perhaps you know, people who are miserable in retirement because they did not plan well financially, or because catastrophic illness wiped out savings, energy, and hope. In his story Peter van Lierop tells how he helps to bring renewed hope to hospital patients as a part-time chaplain. Vicki McClelland Johnson tells how she helped two friends in nursing homes by paying their bills, writing their letters, and reading to them. Virginia Mackenzie describes how she volunteered to record books on audiotapes for blind people—for nine years. She didn't "flunk retirement," as Lee Iacocca says he did (1996, p. 50).

The many retirees I interviewed for this book all said that doing volunteer work gave them a sense of fulfillment and increased their own physical, mental, and spiritual health. Since retirement brings more freedom, it can be the most fulfilling and enjoyable time of life. In her story, Rhoda Iyoya says, "I sincerely believe that we prepare ourselves throughout our lifetime for the creative retirement years—when we have more leisure time to do helpful, creative things." Retirement can certainly be a productive time. As the psalmist in the Bible reminds us, we can "still bear fruit in old age" (Psalm 92:14).

The retirement stories in this book were obtained through interviews using both written and oral questions and answers. For a few, only written questions and answers were used.

Nurse to African Babies, Then to American Retirees

MARABELLE TAYLOR

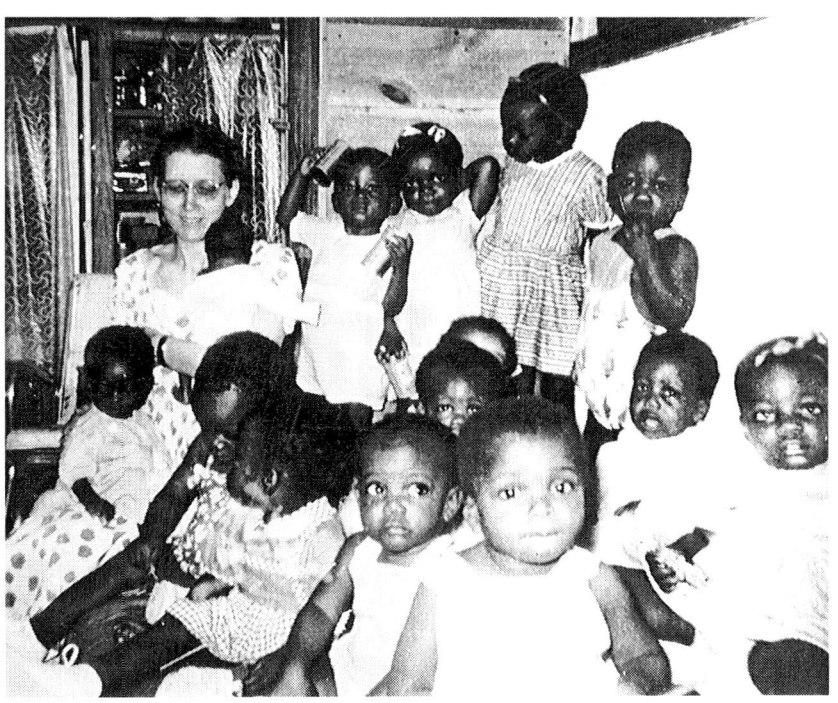

"If we ever lose Marabelle, we will have to hire three people to replace her," said John Rollins. John was speaking as executive director of the retirement and nursing home where Marabelle Taylor serves as a "recycled senior." At age eighty-one, Marabelle is gray-haired and a bit stoop-shouldered, but she seems as active and energetic as ever. She is "recycled" in the sense that she began a new career after retirement, reusing skills developed in an earlier career.

Recently I asked Marabelle to describe a typical day's service for those she assists. She said, "Every day is different for me but I usually help about twelve people with their eyedrops and I pick up their medication at the pharmacy. I drive one or more to a doctor's office or laboratory for treatments—such as chemotherapy or cataract operations. I am in the dining hall for three meals each day as hostess, arranging seating and welcoming guests. Sometimes I have to go and check on someone who doesn't show up for a meal—to see if they are sick or have just forgotten meal time. My day usually begins about 7 a.m. and seldom ends before 10 p.m. And I am on call twenty-four hours a day, seven days a week."

"How do you keep going for such long hours?"

"Well, having been a nurse for about sixty years, I have learned to relieve the pressure by taking short naps in a chair. Now I do that when I have to wait for someone I have taken to a doctor's office."

"How long have you been serving in this retirement ministry?"

"Let me see. I first came here in 1980, when I was a young lady of sixty-five. Now I have been here sixteen years and am age eighty-one."

"How is your own health?"

"Presently I have no health problems. I'm too busy to get sick. Too many people depend on me, and I don't want to let them down. Thankfully, the Lord keeps me going."

"I have seen you taking big packages into the Health Center [Nursing Home]. What's in those big packages?"

"Usually the big packages are special protective 'briefs' for incontinent people, but I also take small packages of medicine as well. Patients in the Health Center can't get out to buy things, so I may even buy some needed clothing or other things for them."

"What is the most difficult part of your medical ministry?"

"Well, it is difficult to see some patients suffering for so long—when they really want to be released from suffering and go on to heaven. Sometimes I find myself praying that the Lord will take someone who is in pain and wants the Lord to end it. When I go, I want to go quickly!"

"Do you get a sense of fulfillment from helping so many people?"

"I certainly do. It is always satisfying to know I am helping people who need me—perhaps making life a little easier for them."

"How long do you think you can keep up this strenuous schedule? At age eighty-one you must be feeling the strain, and want to rest."

"That's in the hands of the Lord. I hope I can keep it up for a while longer. My work is meaningful and enjoyable. And it certainly agrees with me—since I stay in such good health."

"Is this the most difficult part of your entire ministry as a Christian nurse?"

"Oh no. At one time as a nurse in Africa's Cameroon, it was much more stressful. I took my mobile clinic to needy isolated people in the Babimbi Hills. I also helped to care for African babies whose mothers had died, or couldn't feed them, and I was their only hope. I even had to drive a whole day's journey to buy canned milk or dried milk to keep them alive. Once I, and the African girls I hired to help me, took care of thirty-five babies in my home at one time. Another time I had eight babies under age three months to care for in my home, which kept me up a lot at night. When I was not away for clinic work, I worked hard to care for those babies. That was much more demanding than what I do now. But, in twenty years, we saved the lives of three hundred ninety-eight babies."

"Are there any 'fun times' or humorous interchanges with patients to ease the constant pressure? I have heard rumors of humor now and then."

"Oh yes. Bob Taylor wrote some humorous 'nursing home rhymes' about the problems he had in our Health Center. I remember one that went like this: 'Hickory dickory docks / I can't put on my socks. Will someone please send / A nurse who can bend?'

"Mrs. Ada Woodberry retained her sense of humor even at age one hundred two. One morning in our Health Center she refused her breakfast tray saying, 'I don't need to eat breakfast. I'm going to heaven today.' But when the nurse started to take the tray away Ada said, 'Leave the coffee. I will drink it along the way.'"

Millie Brown is one of the people Marabelle takes to doctors for chemotherapy. When I told Millie that John Rollins had said we would have to hire three people to replace Marabelle if we lost her, Millie said, "John is wrong about that. If we ever lose Marabelle, we won't need three people to replace her—we will need *five*."

But I don't want to give the impression that Marabelle has no weaknesses. At her own admission, Marabelle has so little time to care for her apartment that it gets a little messy. That is because with Marabelle, other people's needs come first. But she does have a good sense of humor about her messy apartment. For a while she had a cartoon on her door saying, "I know my apartment is a mess, so next year I am going to *remuddle* it."

Caregiving for an Alzheimer's Spouse

BOB LAZEAR

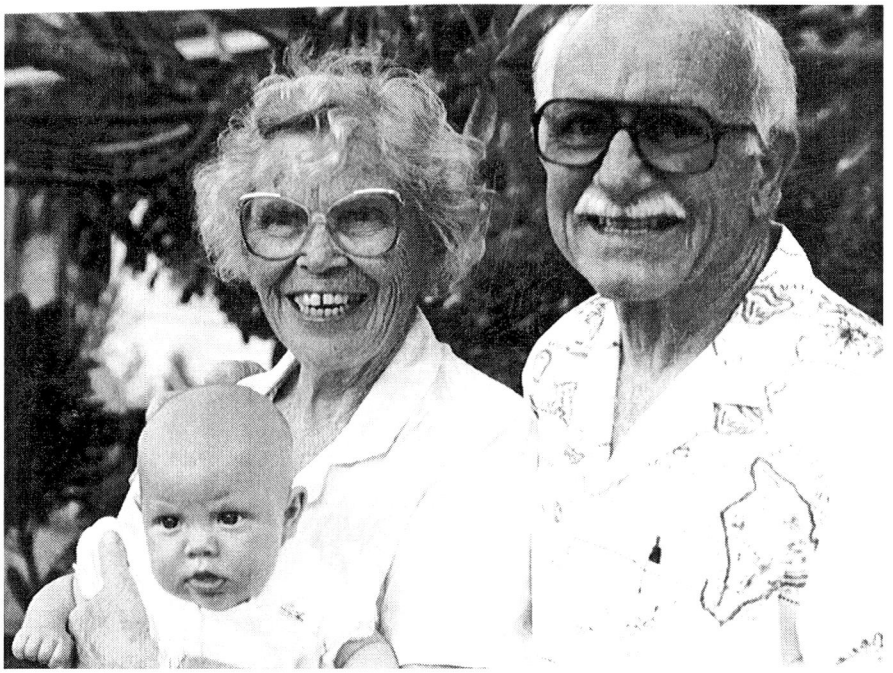

"*Bob, I know your retirement ministry has included serving in six interim pastorates—highlighted by serving one year at the unique Community Church in Madrid, Spain. But, for me, your most remarkable retirement ministry has been the faithful, devoted way you care for your wife, Eleanor, who has <u>Alzheimer's disease</u>.* It must be difficult and painful to see Eleanor gradually lose the ability to take care of herself. Wasn't she all right during your thirty years of missionary service in Colombia?*"

---

*Underlined terms can be found in the Glossary at the end of the book.

"Yes. Eleanor gave piano and voice lessons in Colombia and helped with church choirs. She also taught physical education and English at the High School in Bogotá where I taught Bible and was Chaplain. She still plays the piano a bit, but it is painful to see she has lost most of her skills." Bob's usual cheery smile vanished as a dark shadow of pain chased it away.

"*I remember Eleanor's friend Gene Clark saying, 'Eleanor has the most pleasing voice of anyone I know when she sings hymns.' I also remember her missionary colleague, Betty Wilmot, saying, 'Eleanor was always cooking, sewing, knitting, painting—and she even learned weaving. Then she shared the fruits of her talents with her friends.'*"

"Those good memories of Eleanor's past service for the Lord and his people help to keep me going. And the encouragement of our many friends is a blessing, as I try to care for her now."

"*When did Eleanor begin having problems?*"

"Well, I first noticed them when we were living in Colorado Springs about six or seven years ago. I remember how puzzled I was once when we went camping and Eleanor forgot to bring along several things we needed. That was not like her. She had always been so well organized."

"*I am amazed to see how cheerful and outgoing she seems to be. When I pass by your house, she smiles and waves in a very friendly way, sometimes saying 'Hi' and sometimes just laughing a delighted little laugh.*"

"Yes, but at other times she can get frustrated and stubborn, when I try to protect her by preventing her from wandering off and getting lost."

"*I can understand that. One of my Alzheimer's friends used to try to forcefully take the car keys away from his wife, even after driving became impossible for him. He couldn't understand that his wife was only trying to protect him from hurting himself or someone else.*"

"Yes. That is one of the hardest parts of caregiving: having a loved one get upset and angry with us because they cannot understand our attempts to help and protect them."

"*Do you have to take any special measures to protect Eleanor?*"

"Yes. When I am doing something else and can't watch her carefully, I have to lock the doors so she won't wander off. When I am preparing meals, I sometimes take the telephone off the hook to avoid that distraction."

"Are there times when she seems like her former alert self?"

"Sometimes. Recently our friend, Tom Grubbs, jokingly said to her, 'Eleanor, are you taking good care of this young man?' (meaning me). She laughed and said, 'I'm trying to.' She sounded like her former joke-loving self. I'm sure every Alzheimer's patient and every caregiver is different, but we have good times and bad times. In the bad times, Eleanor can't talk or act reasonably. That hurts."

"I admire the way you manage to care for Eleanor, in spite of the nerve problem that hampers your own walking. I also admire your ability to keep your sense of humor under the daily pressure you endure."

"If I don't laugh sometimes, I will end up crying most of the time. Recently Katie Turner provided a good laugh when she said, 'I don't have to worry about getting Alzheimer's—that happens only to *smart* people.'"

"What are you learning through this caregiving experience?"

"I am learning four important things. First, I am learning that Christ is giving me a new calling. God has spoken to me through I Timothy 5:8 saying, '. . . anyone who won't care for his own relatives when they need help, especially those living in his own family, has no right to say he is a Christian' [Living Bible]. For me these words have meant the Call of God to the *vocation* of caring for my wife, being concerned about all the aspects of her life. Eleanor requires my care during the twenty-four hours of each day. (I have to do all the cooking, wash our clothes, help Eleanor get dressed in the morning, give her the pills she is taking, etcetera, etcetera).

"Second, I am learning that Christ himself identifies with me. At present my wife does not have the use of her powers of reasoning and I can no longer converse with her about the many things we used to talk about. It is a great consolation to me to know that Christ understands, identifying with me, and being concerned about me. He identifies with us to such an extent that he says, 'Come unto me. . . . Take my yoke upon you and learn from me. . . . I will give you rest. . . .' (Mt. 11:28-30). He invites us to be yoked with him, knowing that he will go along teaching us and that he himself will carry a good part of the weight of the yoke, giving us only the weight we can bear.

"The third thing I am learning is that since Christ is with me day by day, I shouldn't worry. We are to live one day at a time, not being concerned about yesterday and not worrying about tomorrow. Christ says, '. . . don't be anxious about tomorrow. God will take care of your tomorrows, too. Live one day at a time (Mt. 6:34 [Living Bible]). Another comforting Bible promise is 'As your days, so shall your strength be' (Deut. 33:25). These are vital lessons I am learning from Christ, the 'Teacher of Afflictions.'

"The fourth lesson is that Christ is teaching me patience, the most difficult lesson to learn and put into practice. My wife is happy most of the time, but sometimes she gets angry and disturbed. What patience is needed! Eleanor is restless and as a result constantly picks up whatever she happens to see, moving things from one place to another without rhyme or reason and often 'hiding' them. How often I have to look for something that is 'lost'! All this requires calm, understanding, love, and above all, patience. Little by little, I am learning patience.

"The words in Colossians 1:11 mean much to me: 'May you be strengthened with all power, according to his glorious might, for all endurance and *patience* with joy. . . .'

"I don't understand what is happening, nor why, but by God's grace I am learning to deal with it, knowing that someday God will show me *the whole big picture* from his vantage point."

The Flower Lady

ELEANOR JAMISON

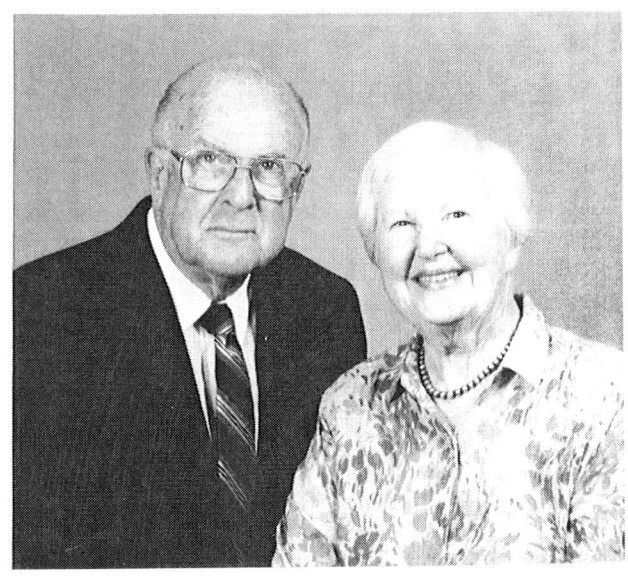

"*I understand some people call you 'The Flower Lady.' How did you get that name?*"

"It grew out of my service to patients in a nursing home. I began that service to ease the pain of losing my own mother. I was devastated when my mother died about the same time I retired from teaching many years in a Head Start program for underprivileged preschoolers. My mother had been in good health, still alert, active, and very much a part of my life. I felt cheated out of giving the loving attention to her that I had pictured as she would age and need more care.

"Missing the contact with the older generation, I began weekly visits with patients in a local nursing home. I gathered baby food jars and put in them tiny bouquets from our garden. That became an opener for a bit of conversation as I took one of the bouquets in to each patient down the hall. Some enjoyed a longer visit as I sat on the edge of their bed. To them I was 'The Flower Lady'—and they filled a void for me. I visited with these dear people for several years." Eleanor's voice was cheerful and upbeat as she shared these things with me, reliving that joyful time of service to others.

"*What was your next project?*"

"I became a grandma, and my family became my central interest again. I loved being a grandma—from holding and rocking to cutting and pasting, to card games and board games, to doll houses and kickball. I provided our home with cribs and high chairs. I baby-sat at our house and theirs. I went to all the school open-houses and the band recitals. But they grow up, and grandmas are not quite as essential as before. It was time for new things."

"*What was the first 'new thing?'*"

"I took up genealogy. It became a fascinating hobby. I got reacquainted with libraries, did research by mail and by travel. I learned to use a computer. I discovered distant 'cousins by the dozens.' I collected books and [photocopied] pages that overflowed my file cabinets and bedrooms. I joined genealogy groups and gave volunteer time in specialized libraries—and I made new friends. And now, fifteen years later, I am still at it."

"*What do you do for exercise?*"

"I love walking. A friend and I still walk briskly a half hour each weekday morning, weather permitting. We have kept this up for seventeen years. Also, since my husband Frank so thoroughly enjoys golf, I took a few golf lessons myself. I don't think my husband ever worried that I would beat him, but I enjoyed the game with friends for several years—until my back told me to quit.

"On a less strenuous level I have always had some kind of handwork in progress—knitting, sewing, and needlepoint. Then a group of us got started on quilting. And now for many years we have been meeting in one another's homes to work on our quilts, or our individual current projects."

"*Have you done volunteer work in your church—you and Frank?*"

"Oh yes. Our church, Arcadia Presbyterian, has been the nucleus for meaningful work for both my husband and myself. We have served as officers in our 'Mariners' group, and I was a deacon at one time. But now, because of my hearing problem, I don't get involved in large group meetings. Yet I still find many jobs to do in my church, such as helping to serve meals to seniors in our dining hall after worship on Sunday and, once a week, I help to straighten up the pew racks in the sanctuary, keeping them in order. Frank and I also contact church members in need and offer to help them any way we can."

"Have you done any community service work?"

"Recently I joined a volunteer group tutoring youngsters in a local elementary school," responded Eleanor. "We are assigned one child with whom we work one day a week for eight weeks. We help with their reading, spelling—or whatever their need."

"Have you tried any educational projects for yourself since retirement?"

"Oh yes. About twelve years ago my husband Frank and I discovered <u>Elderhostels</u>. It's hard to describe how much we've enjoyed attending these week-long classes in interesting locations. During the class in Virginia, we visited Civil War sites and I got a personal insight into our nation's tragic history at that time. Another outstanding class was one on the life and work of Abraham Lincoln, led by a fascinating professor from the University of Arizona. I gained an appreciation of how Lincoln struggled to hold our nation together at a difficult time, and overcome the evil and divisive slave problem.

"At a class in Cambria, California, we studied the life and writings of John Steinbeck, as he wrote about the social problems of our nation in his books, *The Grapes of Wrath* and *Cannery Row.* In twelve years we have attended twenty-three Elderhostels in various states: Arizona, Minnesota, Montana, and Oregon, in addition to California and Virginia. Every one has been a unique experience. We can continue learning."

"How do you find time and energy to do all these things? I am getting exhausted just listening to all you do!"

Eleanor laughed and said, "To tell the truth, at age seventy-eight, I am beginning to run out of steam. I must slow down soon. But, thankfully, the good Lord has blessed me with health and energy. And I hope to keep serving the Lord and his people as long as possible."

Telephone Helpline and Shelter for Battered Women

NANNIE HEREFORD

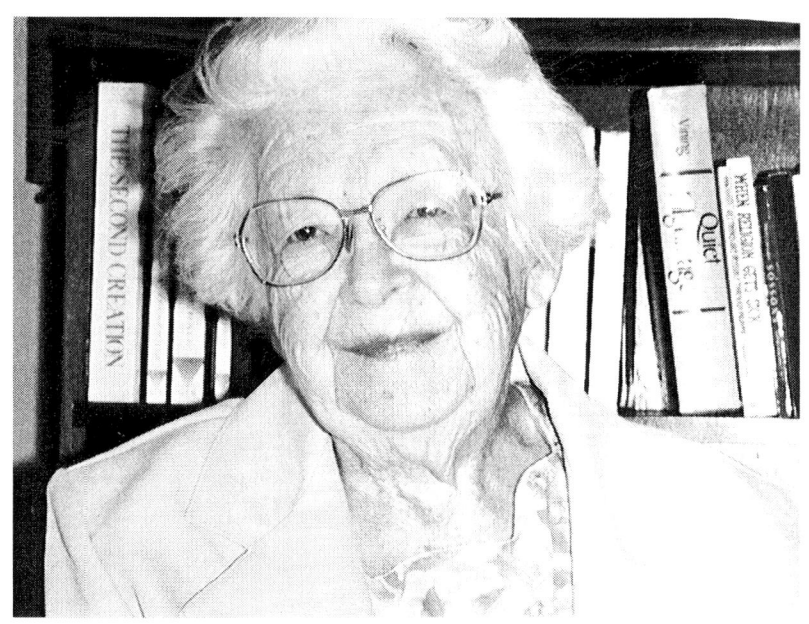

"Nannie, I know that during your last assignment as a missionary to Japan you worked with two Christian groups, one of which became a church. Didn't you also do some work in Tokyo after retiring from church work?"

"Yes," replied Nannie Hereford, brushing back her wavy white hair. "I agreed to teach English for two years at a church-related school there, if I could find an apartment close enough to walk to the school. I am brave but not brave (or foolish) enough to fight Tokyo's commuter traffic every day. After two years, I retired and arranged to stay and work in Tokyo. But after one year I decided to return to the U.S.A. and retire in Nashville, Tennessee."

"*Why did you choose Nashville for retirement?*"

"My single sister, Julia, lived there. She had been my closest family member since my parents' death, so it was natural that I retire near her. Both of us were born in Japan. Our parents were missionaries."

"*What volunteer work did you do in Nashville?*"

"Hating war. One group I worked hard for was Peace Links, started by Betty Bumpers, wife of Senator Bumpers of Arkansas. I arranged monthly meetings, and some special meetings, at my church. Sometimes we met at the local Jewish temple. One year we entertained three women from the Soviet Union, working to promote peace between our two countries. Betty Bumpers still keeps in touch with me, thanking me for helping Peace Links.

"Another important volunteer activity was my work with the Nashville Crisis Center. I had done telephone helpline work in Tokyo and had received extensive training. The Crisis Center welcomed my offer to assist in their helpline work, not only because of my experience and training but also because I was willing to work at night. Being single, I had more control over my schedule than those with families. Sometimes drunks called in and babbled on, but we listened. We knew that everyone who called might be a troubled person who needed someone to listen to them, and we tried to help each one.

"Perhaps the most exciting, and meaningful, help I was able to give came early one Saturday morning. I answered a call from a young woman who said there were eighteen of them who had fled a burning apartment building in their night clothes, barefooted. They were at a neighbor's apartment. They had coffee to drink but were hungry and cold. No one had any money with them, not even a checkbook. She said she had called the Red Cross and the confused person on duty said, 'Call back on Monday.' I assured the girl I would do some calling for her.

"I called Goodwill Industries and they donated some clothing they usually sell. My companion that day was a young dentist. He had served on the Red Cross Board and knew some top officers. He began working on them and the Red Cross finally came up with a two hundred dollar coupon for a department store. I found in our files who was due to serve hot meals to the hungry that day. They agreed that at 1 p.m. they would bring enough cooked spaghetti to the apartment to feed all eighteen hungry people waiting there. I felt good about helping those eighteen people."

"*Didn't you also help some foreigners to learn English as a second language while in Nashville?*"

"Yes. At first I volunteered to help the English as a Second Language classes at Vanderbilt Divinity School for no pay. Those classes were operated by the public school system under [the] Adult Education [program]. The next year I decided that though I was age sixty-seven, I should do some work of economic value. I started teaching four hours a week at three dollars an hour. I continued to teach these classes for about nine years. Inflation raised my pay to twelve dollars an hour. Some of the students were wives of university students or doctors doing research at the hospital. Others were refugees from Vietnam, Laos, and Cambodia. I gained a lot of satisfaction teaching those students, including helping them to understand the Tennessee accent. And I proved I could still 'earn' a paycheck!"

"*Did you do any other volunteer work in Nashville?*"

"Yes. I not only delivered meals on wheels to shut-in people, I also did some work with the American Association of University Women (AAUW) there. My sister Julia was a member and introduced me to the group. I was asked to be the chairperson of the Legislative Committee of this AAUW group. The committee met monthly at my apartment. Often we took postcards to the meetings, asking the members to write legislators about some important issue.

"Also, in cooperation with the Bread for the World group there, we worked to try to remove the sales tax on food—which was a heavy burden to poor people. Tennessee has no state income tax and relies heavily on sales taxes for revenue. We worked hard but didn't succeed. Unlike California, which has no tax on food, Tennessee still taxes food. However, Bread for the World did eventually help to convince the federal government to stop sales taxes on food stamps. I worked on several other legislative issues and was honored by the legislature there when I left Tennessee, but I feel I was not a successful lobbyist."

"*Were there other groups you worked with in Nashville?*"

"Yes. One organization that I worked with, that Julia was not active in, was Church Women United (<u>CWU</u>). Dorothy Copple invited me to join the Social Service Committee of CWU. We sponsored many projects. One year we took over an old house no longer fit for human habitation. We remodeled it, painted it, and put in new tiling and fixtures in the bathroom. The next year Dorothy Copple said, 'We need a new, long-term project to work on, any suggestions?'

"I said, 'At the Crisis Center the biggest problem I hear on the Helpline is the women who are battered by their husbands, but they have no place to run to get away from him. We need a woman's emergency shelter. After some discussion we agreed that would be a good project. We started with small individual gifts. Then I began to put pressure on our local <u>Presbytery</u> (organized group of Presbyterian churches) asking the leaders to help us. Although not a member of [the] Presbytery, I attended every meeting where our request was to be considered. Finally, knowing I would give them no peace until they helped, they voted to give seven thousand dollars. Later, they doubled this to fourteen thousand dollars. Encouraged by this I put the squeeze on the leaders of my local church and they gave one thousand dollars. Eventually, our Church Women United group raised a total of thirty thousand dollars.

"At first we rented a house as a shelter (for one dollar a year) but became able to buy one. The YWCA took over the operation of the Haven House. God blessed the project and it continues to rescue <u>battered women</u> today."

"*Have you done any traveling since retirement?*"

"Yes. In the summer of 1980, my three sisters and I joined a tour to Oberammergau, Germany to see the famous Christian *Passion Play* there. Since moving to California, I attend an annual family reunion in Tennessee, and usually visit my sister, Grace, in Ohio at the same time."

"*Why did you move from Nashville to your present place of retirement here in California?*"

"Well, after my sister Julia died, there was no family left in Nashville. I decided to settle down at Westminster Gardens in

California, where I still had two nephews living nearby. I had been in Nashville eleven years, from 1974 to 1985."

"*What volunteer work have you done here?*"

"One volunteer project developed out of the church I joined in Arcadia, California. Through the church I helped with the organization of an agency to give food and other help to the homeless and families in need. It was called Interfaith Community Outreach (IFCO). After it moved from our church to another city, I continued to help gather and distribute food but finally stopped. Amazingly, they managed to get along without me!"

"*Have you had hobbies to relieve the pressure of your many activities? I am amazed at how you keep so active and independent at age eighty-eight.*"

"Oh yes. In Nashville I volunteered to lead a Canasta club at the local Senior Center and enjoyed playing on Friday morning, followed by lunch together. Here I am part of a bridge club meeting on Tuesday evenings. I love music and attended many concerts with Julia, and now with friends here. I also love to read books and see good dramas."

"*How is your health now? I remember trying to help you recently and you said, 'No! I can do that myself!'*"

"At age eighty-eight, my general health is pretty good, except for declining eyesight. By using a reading machine, I can still do a little reading and writing, but I am legally blind. I live alone in my own apartment and can take care of most of my own needs. But I do eat my meals in the dining hall here and get help in cleaning my apartment. When I forget something, my friends kindly say 'join the club,' since our average age here is eighty-one and we all are good 'forgetters.' And, like others, I have to push myself to keep going, but I want to stay independent as long as possible.

"I hear that playing bridge helps to avoid Alzheimer's disease, and I am determined to keep playing until my partners give up on me. So far, so good!

"Thankfully, the Lord has blessed me with a long and meaningful life, and I am proud to be as active and independent as I am at my age. I am slowing down but, as one retiree here said, 'I ain't dead yet.' And I thank God for the promise of each new day."

The Library Lady

MARY RUTH HOYT

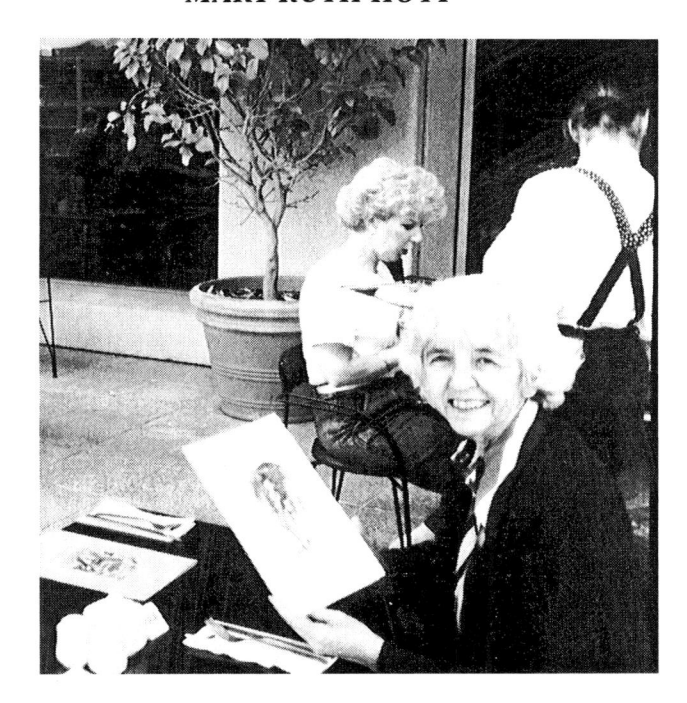

"*Mary Ruth, when I first met you in Maryville, Tennessee in 1973 you were already working for ALCOA (Aluminum Company of America). How long did you work there?*"

"Let me see. I began there in 1943 and retired in 1985. That means I worked there for about forty-two years—quite a good record there when compared to today's volatile job market." There was a note of pride in her strong, husky voice.

"*What were your specific duties there?*"

"I did many things. But most of the time I was an administrative assistant in a Production Department. I worked out schedules for about five hundred people, kept the personnel records of those employees, and I fed daily rate changes and other personnel information into the computer. The computer, at first, was a new-fangled contraption I learned to use—beyond the older typewriter and copying machines I began with. [laughs]

"I also had to know every detail of the Union Contract, and do any jobs that came my way. Once, during an employee strike, I even briefly took over a truck driver's job—helping to haul away trash and garbage that had piled up on our grounds. I got kidded about that. Thankfully, I didn't wreck the dump truck.

"Although we joked a lot, I had a good relationship with both management and the hourly employees. I really enjoyed my work."

"*How did you plan for retirement?*"

"Well, after observing a number of people who were unhappy, or even bitter, about being forced to retire—or demoted near the end of their careers—I decided I would 'call the shots' about my retirement. So in the year I reached age sixty-two (which was as soon as I could retire), I approached my boss a little early and requested retirement.

"He asked me to continue working, unless I was really determined to retire that year. I agreed to stay on a while longer. Before reaching my next birthday, I knew it was time to retire. I had the 'right mind-set.' I left the company feeling good about everything, and I have never regretted my decision."

"*Although living alone, you decided to stay in your own home, didn't you?*"

"Yes. There is a good retirement home in the community with a nursing home connected to it, but I hope I will never have to go there. That kind of life does not appeal to me. I'm too independent."

"*After hearing about all the library work you have been doing, I now think of you as 'The Library Lady.' How did you get started in library work?*"

"I joined a group called Friends of the Library and was the treasurer there. And I have done a lot of volunteer work at our local library. I now work on a regular basis, one day a week. Being single, I have the time."

"*What do you do there?*"

"I shelve books and help patrons, but when other jobs occur, I also volunteer for special needs. I have always loved reading. I have often thought that if I were doing my education over again, I would get a library degree—but I waited too long."

"Didn't you also do some volunteer work at the local hospital?"

"Yes. I helped to deliver newspapers to patients' rooms. But it was hard to see so many people suffering there, and I couldn't help them."

"But you did help an elderly friend, didn't you?"

"Oh yes. I had power of attorney for an older friend. She was one of my high school teachers. I did shopping and ran errands for her while she still lived in her apartment. I paid her bills after she went into a nursing home. She had no family, so I became her family substitute. When she was healthier, we enjoyed many good times together—hiking, studying wild flowers, and eating out."

"Aren't you still doing some community service work to help needy people?"

"Yes. I work in the Community Benefit Sales Room at New Providence Church. We process clothing and household items for a monthly rummage sale."

"How do you help there?"

"I help to clean, sort, and price the clothing. Some items are given to people in need—destitute people, low-income people, or people who have lost things when their house burned down. Even the items we sell are priced very low to make it easy for needy people to buy them. And the money we make goes to other charitable agencies in our community."

"What do you do for your own continuing educational and recreational needs?"

"I attend some Elderhostels, here and overseas. And, as you know from the exotic postcards I send out, I love to travel—all over the world. The Elderhostels combine education and travel in a wonderful way. I guess I am a real travel 'junkie' and need to have a travel 'fix' occasionally to keep my inner self refreshed."

"How do you arrange your many travels?"

"Sometimes I go with a tour group, and sometimes friends and I travel on our own. We often rent a car and enjoy visiting out-of-the-way places, here and overseas. It is more challenging when traveling on your own."

"What kind of challenges have you faced?"

"Perhaps the most exciting challenge was daring to go on a hot-air balloon ride over the desert in Southern California. Thankfully, we didn't crash and have to search for water holes to survive."

"Are you still doing volunteer work for your church? As I remember, you did a lot of that when I was serving your church as pastor."

"I still take an active part in women's circle work, sometimes serving as an officer or leader. I also take my turn presenting the Bible lessons. I am an ordained church elder, and I support the activities of the Women's Association."

"Didn't you once serve on the Director's Board of the Sunset Gap Community Service Center?"

"I am just beginning my third term on that Board."

"What are your duties there? I know you give spiritual help."

"I have served as secretary of the Board and am now on the personnel committee. As you know, the Center serves needy people in an isolated mountain area. We have educational and recreational programs for children and adults. And we help provide food and clothing when there is an urgent need."

"How is your own health holding up under this busy schedule? To me you seem almost like a 'superwoman' when I add up all the things you do."

"Thankfully, I have no health problems. But I do try to eat healthful food, walk a lot, and take vitamins and calcium. I also do yard work. Every day I thank the Lord for my blessings. For my spiritual health, I daily use the prayer and meditation booklet, *The Upper Room*. But I must admit I am not a very good meditator. My mind wanders around a little, but I do keep trying. Speaking of my mind wandering, I forgot to mention that I belong to a group called American Association of University Women."

"What do you do with University Women?"

"I have been secretary and treasurer of that group, but now it's more work with books. I am co-chair of the annual book fair. This requires a lot of work—collecting the books, categorizing them, pricing them, and packing them into boxes. This project recirculates books in the community. The money earned helps to provide scholarships for students on the local, national, and international level. It also helps other educational projects.

"The prices are low so people with limited funds can buy them. And the books we cannot sell, we give to the local library for their ongoing sale and to the local community college—which also has a book sale for scholarships."

"What advice would you give a friend preparing for retirement?"

"First, prepare financially. I invested in a tax-free IRA (Individual Retirement Account) plus other investments. You should take an interest in things beyond your own career and hobbies. Don't become a couch potato sitting in front of a TV. And don't become a rocking-chair cowboy, riding aimlessly into a meaningless sunset. Most of all, prepare yourself mentally and spiritually. I did, and I am enjoying every minute of my retirement. God has blessed me, and I am grateful."

Recording Books on Tape for Blind People

VIRGINIA MACKENZIE

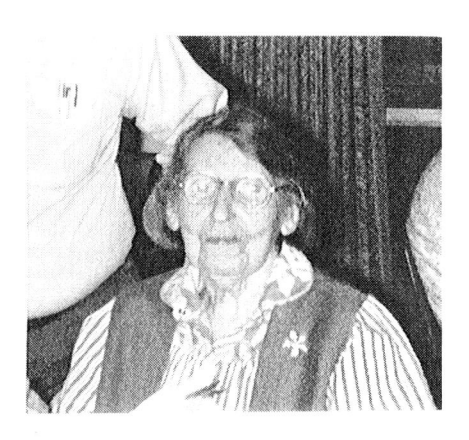

"When did you enter Westminster Gardens Retirement Community?"

"I came here in 1959. Now I have lived here thirty-seven years—longer than any of about two hundred residents. And at age one hundred one, I have outlived many others who came here much later than I did." A smile of pride brightened her face, with its aquiline nose and strong jawline.

"To live so long you must have good eating and exercise habits."

"Well, yes and no. Growing up as a child in Scotland, I did eat plain, simple foods like meat, potatoes, lima beans, and fish, and I have always had a lot of exercise walking. But I never liked some of the so-called health foods such as broccoli, zucchini, and onions. I felt I was in good company when President George Bush said he didn't like broccoli."

"*Someone mentioned to me that you are a 'chocoholic' and want to get your chocolate 'fix' every day. Do you really eat chocolate every day?*"

"Well, I'm not sure I like the 'chocoholic' terminology, but I do eat a little chocolate almost every day. But, unlike one of my friends, I am not tempted to eat a whole box in one sitting. I usually eat only one piece a day."

"*I heard someone say they lived a long time because they 'picked the right parents and grandparents.' Do you think you inherited long-life genes from your Scottish ancestors?*"

"Maybe my sturdy Scotch ancestry deserves some credit, but I have tried to take care of myself—and certainly the Lord deserves the major credit for granting me such a long life and good health."

"*What was life like here at Duarte when you came here thirty-eight years ago?*"

"Well, the Gardens had only about sixty-three people here then, compared to over two hundred now, and we had only two office workers, Dr. Howell Lair as director and Miss Byrd Rice as secretary. I became their volunteer helper in the office."

"*What did you do?*"

"I did many things. I answered the telephone. I helped to put mail in the mail slots for all the residents. And I eventually became responsible for locking all the public doors at night and opening them in the morning. One special door took about thirteen turns of the key to open. I often slept with a bunch of keys under my pillow. Sometimes residents would wake me saying, 'Can you help me? I locked myself out of my apartment.'"

"*I have heard you called the 'keeper of the keys' and also the '7-11' lady. What does the 7-11 mean?*"

"It means that on Saturdays I took over the office duties—going in at 7 a.m. and staying until after 11 a.m. Being single, my schedule was easy to arrange."

"*I also heard that in addition to unlocking office doors, you helped to make tape recordings of books for the benefit of blind people. That way you helped to 'unlock reading doors,' by allowing* them to use their ears instead of their eyes to enjoy a book. How did that get started?"

"Well, that really started while I was teaching in Baiko School in Japan because it was there I got the desire to do so. There I had a blind Japanese friend. I admired her faith and courage in taking care of most of her own needs, even though it was hard to do. I resolved then and there that someday I would do something to help blind people. Then, soon after retiring here I heard on TV that volunteers were needed to record books, and I volunteered."

"How did it work out?"

"It was difficult at first. I had to take a long bus ride, with two transfers, to get to the place in Los Angeles. It took most of my day, once a week. They said my voice was not quite right for recording but they welcomed my offer to work the machine for another person to read. I soon learned my reader, Mrs. Lyle Hoag, lived near me in the Duarte area. Then, for nine years she drove me by car and we recorded together until she had to stop."

"Did you do any other community service work?"

"Oh yes. I was often asked to speak about Japan and life there in nearby elementary schools, including one school for retarded children. Many of the children had fathers, or other relatives, who had served in Japan during World War II—and they were fascinated by my stories about life in Japan. And twice I served as president of our residents' association here. I also wrote the historical records for the Gardens for several years."

"Did you develop any close friendships here at Westminster Gardens? As president of the residents' association, you had a good opportunity."

"Oh yes, I developed many friendships. One of the most active and interesting friendships was with David and Louella Tappan. David was a 'thinker' and Louella was a 'pusher.' She pushed to put her husband's ideas into practice. One project I worked on with them was to get mission speakers for local churches—especially Pasadena Presbyterian Church. I also helped Louella in getting a booklet written about some of the unique work residents had done in the mission field. Louella titled the book *Looking Back*, and it included over thirty stories. David was president of the residents' association when I first came here."

"*I am amazed at how clear your memory is at age one hundred one.*"

"Well, I'm a little amazed myself. It seems I can remember names better now than I could about fifteen years ago when I was eighty-five years young."

"*Maybe you had better will your brain to science so they can try to find out why your memory is so good at your age.*"

"Well, I don't know about that. They might find some things there that I don't want them to know about."

"*All of your retirement service has certainly been meaningful. What did you enjoy most in your service for others?*"

"I think recording for blind people was the most meaningful and enjoyable. But I am thankful that the Lord enabled me to do all those things. And I am also grateful that, unlike my Alzheimer's disease friends, my mind is still clear and I can get about a little using my walker. I never have used that rocking chair I bought when I first retired."

Author's Note:

On a sad note, Virginia MacKenzie is no longer able to see well enough to read or write. But she is benefitting from others who volunteer to do what she once did.

A "Can't Say No" Volunteer

JUNE HANSEN

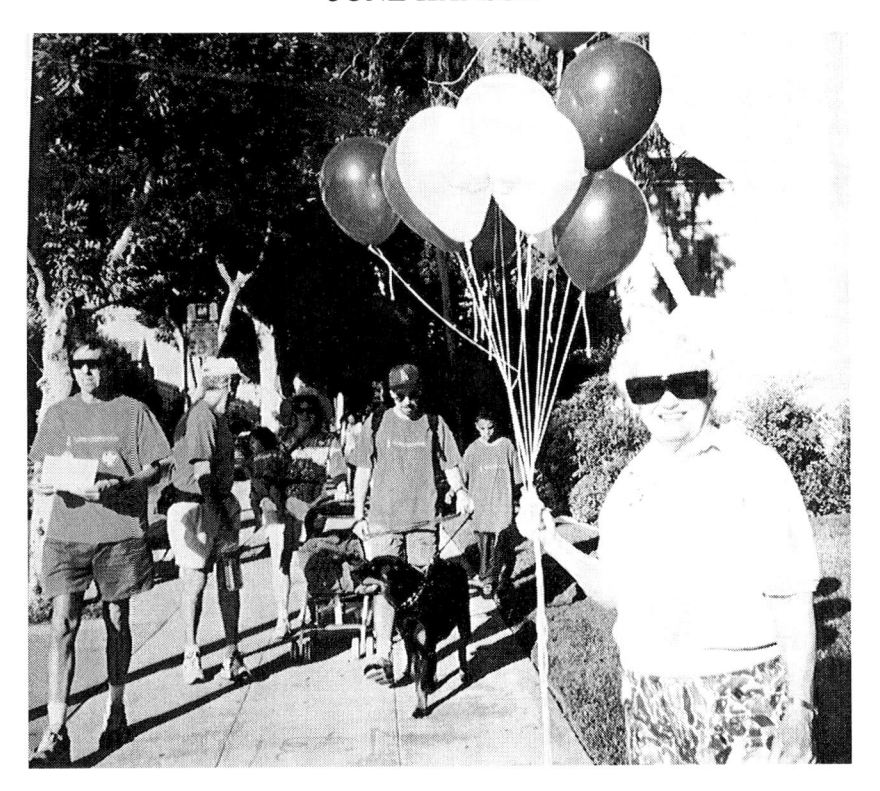

"*June, I know many active volunteers but I think you are the most active volunteer I have ever met. In fact, you have done so many things I'm not sure I can name them all.*" As June listened to me, a sunny smile brightened her jolly round face.

"You don't have to name them. [laughs] The YWCA here in Pasadena has conveniently named them for you. The YWCA honored me as a volunteer over a year ago and listed my volunteer activities. Let me show you that list."

Taking the list she pulled from a file I read, "June Hansen is known for more than fifty years of supporting and fundraising work for the Visually Handicapped, the Girl Scouts (a troop leader for twelve years), Presbyterian Homes for the Aged, March of Dimes, Union Station's work with homeless people, International Visitors Program, and the YWCA. For her work with the Y program at Camp Bluff Lake she won the title, or nickname, 'Mother Pine Cone.'

"She was also PTA President at Washington Elementary School and on the Board of Noyes Elementary Schools. She was President of the Women's 'Sisterhood' called PEO and the Fidelia Club for teacher's wives."

"Wow! That's quite a list of volunteer jobs. How did you get involved in so many things?"

"Well, when there is a need I just can't say no. But nearing my eightieth birthday, I simply must learn to say no soon."

"Have you always lived here in the Pasadena, California area?"

"Oh no. I was born in Lake Forest, Illinois, and reared in Racine, Wisconsin. I moved to Pasadena after I married my husband, Alfred in 1943, and he was sent for military service in the South Pacific. We moved to this Altadena home in 1955, and have now lived in this same house for forty-one years."

"Where did you work before retirement?"

"I have never really 'retired.' I worked for a time in personnel at the Broadway Department Store and with the famous 'Manhattan Project' at Cal-Tech. During the World War II years, I did secretarial and clerical work. I do like to write, but I must confess I was never too fond of being a 'secretary.'"

"What volunteer work have you done with your church?"

"Many things. Church work is a pleasure for me. I taught Sunday School at Pasadena Presbyterian Church (PPC) for over twenty years. I served as an elder twelve years, was president of our Women's Association—and it was a joy to be a 'commissioner' to the <u>general assembly</u> of our National Church when they met in Atlanta in 1993. I was proud to be there when the northern and southern streams of our Presbyterian Church U.S.A. joined hands and hearts and became one church. And can you believe that at age eighty I just agreed to become <u>moderator</u> of our Women's Program again at my local church!

"My husband, in spite of some health problems, is a valued member of our church choir but, for some strange reason, no one wants me to sing!"

"Have you always been a Presbyterian?"

"Oh no. I was baptized a Lutheran, joined the Methodist Church in my early teens, and during the war years—1943 to 1947—I attended a Baptist church with a friend with whom I worked.

"I really wanted to go to Pasadena Presbyterian Church then, but I decided I had better not take any unnecessary risks. A sign in front of the Presbyterian church said, 'Welcome to all Service Men!' As a lonely new bride, with my husband away for military service, I felt I shouldn't expose myself to the temptation of seeing all those handsome men in uniform on a regular basis.

"My husband, Al, returned home after the war. Then, with him by my side, I could resist all temptation. We started going to Pasadena Presbyterian and have now worshipped and served there for almost fifty years.

"When Union Station (program of food and shelter for homeless men, women, and children) was housed at the Congregational Church in Pasadena, Al and I supervised the twenty-eight beds in a large hall—where we fed the needy supper, talked with them, and took them to the showers before bedtime at 11 p.m. Supervising the women I was sometimes asked to pray for them. As we got better acquainted, they even allowed me to pray for them as they showered behind closed curtains—not seeing it as an invasion of their privacy.

"Our cots were right in the midst of the guests, and we'd hear the deep breathing, coughing, and snoring in their often restless sleep. When some children were there, I really worried that they would not get enough sleep."

"How is your health after all these years of hard work?"

"For an eighty-year-old, my health is okay. I realize I have problems remembering names of people, plants, and possessions—where is my brain? I lose it frequently—but since most friends my age also forget things, I blend right in with the senior citizens around me.

"Amazingly, even the young Girl Scouts I led many years ago are now past age fifty. My advice to them is to think not in terms of retirement but in terms of how they can serve God and others as long as they live. Thankfully, some continue to ask for my advice—making me still feel needed in my old age.

"This last year I have taken responsibility for trying to find volunteers for the Habitat for Humanity project in Duarte. As you may know, they provide homes for people who could otherwise not afford them. How disappointing it was when some people refused to help saying they were 'retired'—that is the best way to truly begin growing 'old.' Thankfully, I did find some who not only volunteered their help but did so joyfully."

"I helped with that project a little myself. And thanks to you, and others who helped, a friend of mine is moving into one of those eight new Habitat homes. He is Juan Aguilar, a cook in our dining hall at Westminster Gardens retirement community. He, his wife, and three charming young daughters expect to move in by Easter, just five days from now.

"His family has met the requirements. They don't earn enough to get a conventional loan but do earn enough to eventually pay back the interest-free loan from Habitat. They have put in the required hours of personal labor on the house (called 'sweat equity'). And they are hardworking, trustworthy people."

"I'm glad to hear Juan's family is moving in at Easter. It is an appropriate time for them to begin their new life there. For us Christians, Easter means 'new life'—Christ rising from the dead and preparing the way for our new life in heaven.

"One reason I like the spring season is that I see new life awakening all around me. Just this morning I was working in my garden with new green plants springing up everywhere. I was reminded that it is God's free gifts of sunshine, rain, and fresh air that make all new life possible. My heart filled with joy and I thanked God for all the blessings given to me."

A Retirement Ministry in Twenty-Five Countries

PAUL LINDHOLM

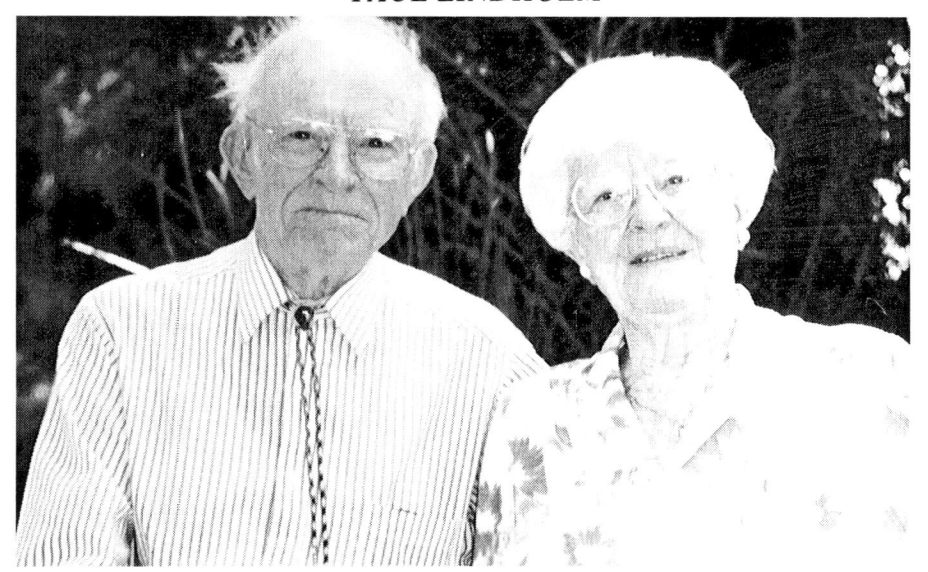

Having heard that after reaching retirement age Paul Lindholm conducted training sessions on Christian giving in over twenty-five countries, I wanted to learn more about his unique retirement ministry.

"How difficult is it to teach the basic principles of Christian giving in other cultures?"

Paul's sun-browned face and sparkling eyes lit up as he began telling me his fascinating mission story. "Well, it is always a challenge. After I spoke about giving in a church in Mexico the choir director asked, 'Do you think a person can be a Christian without giving?' I responded with another question: 'Do you think a person can be a Christian without loving?' The immediate reply was, 'Certainly not. The Great Commandment is you must love God with all your heart.' I then continued, 'Could a husband or a wife love each other without giving to the other?' The response was immediate, 'Impossible.' The choir director then agreed that the question had been answered."

"Did you learn of any good examples of giving in your travels?"

"Once a Filipino doctor who was treasurer of his church told me about a poor employee at his hospital. Sometimes scheduled to work on Sundays, she would give her weekly offering to him to take to the worship service. One week, in addition to her regular offering, she came with an unexpectedly large offering for typhoon victims on a nearby island. 'That's too much for you to give,' the kind doctor said, taking from his pocket an equal amount he said he would give that for her. When she started crying the doctor said, 'I'm trying to help you!' She shook her head and finally was able to say, 'You're taking from me the greatest joy I have in my life.'"

"Did you find any examples of people giving their time and talents instead of money?"

"Oh yes. One Sunday in a mountain village in the Philippines, twenty-three people were received into church membership. A friend of mine was there and the pastor explained to him that seventeen of the twenty-three had been led to Christ by one man, who walked many miles to visit in their homes. Imagine my friend's surprise when he met the man after the service and found that one of his legs was swollen to twice the size of the other. How could he walk those rough mountain trails?

"'You must go to the hospital to get that leg attended to,' my friend advised. 'You seem to have a bad case of <u>elephantiasis</u>, which needs immediate care.'

"Quickly came the response, 'Yes, I plan to do that soon, but first I am waiting for three more families that I am visiting to come to the Lord.' He was risking his own health to help those he felt had spiritual needs greater than his own physical needs."

"Did you learn about any Christians facing danger, or overcoming superstitions, to help others?"

"In one isolated village, I led a worship service in the home of the police chief. He had been won to Christ because when his pregnant wife died, the Christian women were the only ones who would prepare her for burial. The non-Christian women feared the taboo that said their children would be born dead if they touched a dead pregnant woman.

"That act of love and courage not only led the police chief to the Lord but also led him to use his own home for worship services."

"*Do you remember any other good deeds done by Christian women?*"

"Let me share with you the story of how a wife finally won her husband to the Lord in an unusual way. Even though he never attended church, she did persuade him to give the money to buy a small organ needed by her church. Then, wanting to see how his gift was being used, he started coming to church—and eventually became a Christian. As Jesus said, 'Where your treasure is, there will your heart be also' (Mt. 6:21). This man's heart had followed his 'treasure.'"

"*I understand you have published two books since retirement. What were they about?*"

"The first book, *Shadows from the Rising Sun*, was about hiding in the Philippine mountains when Japan occupied that country during World War II, while I was a missionary co-worker there. The second book, *First Fruits*, is a book about Christian giving—which grew out of my many years of teaching about giving."

"*When was the* First Fruits *book published?*"

"It was published in 1993, when I was age eighty-nine."

"*You have certainly 'borne fruit in old age,' as the Bible says in Psalm 92:14. How old were you when you last worked with people from another country?*"

"Well, I still work with a Filipino group here, but my last mission trip was teaching stewardship in a seminary in Guatemala when I was a young man of seventy-six.

"In Ethiopia I learned that 'old age' means different things there. Their life expectancy is still about age forty-five, and when I was there thirty-two years ago, it was even lower. When an Ethiopian man learned I was then age sixty he said, 'Mr. Lindholm, you are now an *old man*! Who will carry on your present work?' I wonder what that man would say if he knew that thirty-two years later, at age ninety-two, I still help out at a Filipino church near here. I supervise the elders' meetings."

"*What kind of responses have you received when teaching about Christian giving?*"

"Well, after doing my best to teach Christian giving to one group, a man came up to me and said, 'If churches use your material on giving, it will stir up some of them a bit. I must confess that I have been shook up a bit myself.' But, since it was God's spirit that shook him up, I can't take credit for it. For me to take credit would be like what the flea said to the elephant. Do you know that story?"

When I said no, Paul continued, "The story goes like this. A small flea was riding on the back of an elephant. When the huge elephant crossed a stream on a suspension bridge, it creaked and swung wildly with every step. Reaching the other side safely, the flea said to the elephant, 'We certainly made that bridge shake, didn't we!'"

"Do you remember any other unusual response to you?"

"There was one interesting one in Ghana. After teaching there a man said to me, 'Get some rest back in your homeland then return here to Ghana with Mrs. Lindholm to work with us some more. I promise you that at the end we'll give you a first-class funeral.'"

Helping Needy People and Prostitute Rescue Work

FAYE SPEER

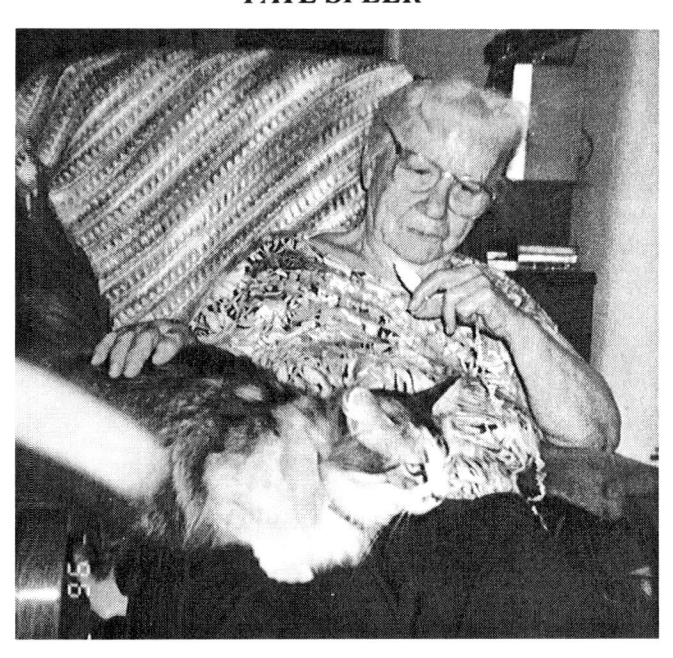

"My wife, Lillian, tells me that you are one of the most active volunteers she knows. But before we get into your volunteer work in retirement, I would like to know what you did before retirement."

"Well," replied cheery and chubby Faye, "for about twenty years I worked for the State of California. I was a claims examiner for the state's disability insurance program. It was my job to see that those who needed, and deserved, disability payments got them—and to prevent fraud when undeserving people tried to rip off the taxpayer for false claims. I was good at it, if I do say so myself."

"*I understand that you have lived in this same house in Baldwin Park for forty-six years. How is California life working out now, as you grow older?*"

"Very well, so far. I lost my husband seventeen years ago, but my four cats are company, my family visits, and I have good neighbors. My cats are named Scat, Flossie, Folly, and Bernice. Scat is so named because she appeared at my back door one day and refused to leave, in spite of my continually telling her to scat. My son, Rich, is with me at the present time. He graduated from Louisville Seminary and is now circulating his 'PIF' [Personal Information Form] to prospective churches that may need a pastor.

"My daughter is far away in Iowa, but she and her husband visit me occasionally. My daughter's three stepchildren make me a happy grandma. Now the stepchildren are getting married and providing more family to enjoy. I love being a grandma."

"*I understand you do a lot of gardening. Is that true?*"

"Yes. I have a large yard with many fruit trees and I have always enjoyed gardening. I usually raise such vegetables as tomatoes, green beans, corn, and squash, and I take care of the fruit from my trees in season. I make jams and jellies as gifts at Christmastime (as well as in between)."

"*Now tell me about your volunteer work—which my wife admires so much.*"

"Well, I'm afraid my life is not very exciting or interesting to others, but I have enjoyed doing quite a bit of volunteer work.

"For a number of years I did volunteer work for the Mary Magdalene Program, a rescue project for prostitutes. They take carefully screened prostitutes into their 'haven house' and seek to rehabilitate them. They help them to recover a sense of self-worth, train them, and help them to find good jobs. I assisted with the fashion shows they put on to raise money for the project. I enjoyed that and got a sense of fulfillment from helping those needy women."

"*Are many of the women really rehabilitated through this program?*"

"Oh, yes. Since we started the program, over one hundred women have been helped to find a better life. I know of only two who relapsed into prostitution. That's a better success rate than might be expected since most of these women came from dysfunctional homes. Most of the rehabilitated ones are helped to find jobs as secretaries or salespersons. But one lovely Caucasian lady I know got a job with the Walt Disney Studios as a cartoonist. Some of these women have latent talents that just need to be developed. One attractive, husky, black woman decided she wanted to go to welding school and is now an effective welder, holding her own among men welders and proving she is worthy of their respect.

"Amazingly, a few rehabilitated mothers have been reunited with children that had to be taken away from them when they were 'street women.' There would be little hope for children reared in that type of destructive atmosphere. The way it is done is through a <u>halfway house</u> provided by the Mary Magdalene Project. This is a place to retrain the women and help them to become good, responsible parents. After the women learn the housekeeping, child care, and financial skills needed for a stable home, they are reunited with their children. It was a joy to see some of them accept Christ as their Lord and Savior."

"*Didn't you also do volunteer work for the 'Food Bank' in West Covina?*"

"Oh yes. I wanted to help in that effort to provide food and other items for needy people. My job was to counsel the needy people who came in for help. I consulted them about the things they might need and then filled a bag with the food, clothing, and other things needed. We had items arranged on shelves and all of us there had certain guidelines to follow. Sometimes our help was the difference which saved them from becoming homeless. Churches and private donations provided most of the funds needed. Some needed things for young children while others had adult needs, but, whatever the need, we tried to help—including spiritual counseling if they needed and wanted that."

"*My wife tells me you do a lot of volunteer work for your local church and the Presbytery [Organized Group of Churches].*"

"Yes. My life has always centered around my church. I have led programs for women in my local church, served on the Session (ruling elders group) and served on so many committees I can hardly remember them all. It is the same with our Presbytery. At present I am Vice Moderator of the 'Governance' Committee of Presbytery. We oversee the records churches keep of membership, attendance at worship and other programs, leadership activities, and all church programs. We also study and make recommendations for making new rules and regulations to guide the National Church work. Currently, I am also serving as an <u>enabler</u> for the Presbyterian Women of our Presbytery.

"But one of the most important volunteer services I have provided for my local church is as 'liaison' person between the Session (elder's group) and our church's thriving Child Care Center. We serve more than ninety children from infants to kindergarten age. We try to provide care, education, and spiritual guidance for the children and their parents. My job is to make sure the elders know what we are doing for the children and try to inspire them to guide and support the Child Care Center in any way they can."

"With all those volunteer activities going on, don't you find it hard to work it all in—or even remember meeting times?"

"Oh yes," said Faye, with her trademark cheery laugh. "Once I was late for a 'governance' committee meeting and someone joked, 'Faye, you need to *govern* your own time schedule better.'"

"Do you have time for any hobbies?"

"Oh, I enjoy reading. I like all kinds of books, adventure, educational, inspirational—you name it—my curiosity knows no limits. I also keep busy with knitting and quilting when not tied up with volunteer work or housework."

"How is your health?"

"At age seventy-nine, I am beginning to feel my age. And I have rather severe arthritis, but in spite of that, I stay active and go to a pool for water exercises two or three times a week. I guess I will finally die with my 'volunteer boots' still on." [laughs]

"If I may ask a very personal question, do you ever worry about dying?"

"Oh no. I am ready to go at any time—but I'm in no hurry. I would like to stick around as long as the Lord has some useful work for me to do. I would hate to miss any of the adventures the Lord still has in mind for me."

Author's Note:

Recently, Faye greeted me with the joyful news that her son, Richard, had accepted a call to serve a local church, and that his ministry is progressing well.

A Retirement Ministry Team

HAL AND KIRBY DAVIS

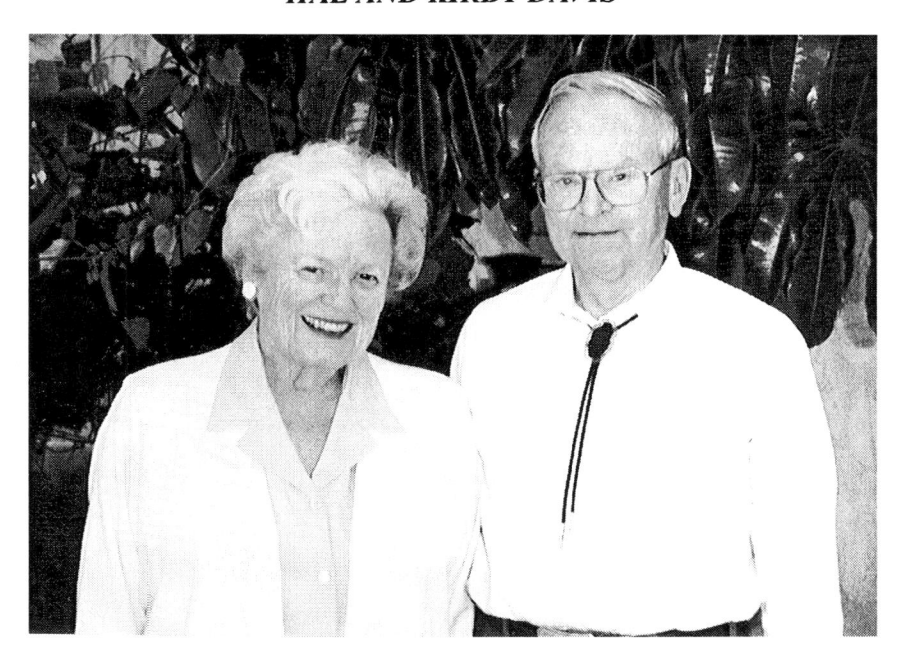

"*Hal, I know that after thirty-nine years of pastoral ministry, you retired in 1989, followed by a part-time position as a parish associate in Lakewood, Colorado. What did you and your wife, Kirby, do at Lakewood?*"

"Well," replied Reverend Harold Davis, "Visiting sick and shut-in people was my chief ministry, and Kirby helped in this. We tried to bring the light of Christ's comfort and healing power to people who were in pain, lonely, or discouraged. We often quoted Jesus' words: 'Come to me, all you who are weary and burdened, and I will give you rest.'" I could feel the love in Hal's warm, strong voice as he told me these things.

"We also organized and coordinated a support group for retired people. Having to face retirement challenges ourselves, we enjoyed sharing our experiences with other retirees—and learning from them. Kirby sang in the choir and helped with the Presbyterian Women's program. For me, it was a half-time position with a half-time salary—which did benefit us."

"When did you come to this retirement community of Westminister Gardens?"

"We sold our home in Westminster, Colorado (near Denver) in June 1992 and came here. Kirby's mother, Wilma Filson, rejoiced to have us join her here. She was age ninety-five at that time. Having both a mother and daughter retired in the same place here is a special distinction we enjoy.

"Kirby's mother, now age ninety-nine, still lives alone in her own apartment, but we do help her with shopping, laundry, and other tasks as needed. It is amazing how she can still do her own cooking and take care of most of her own needs. She is the widow of the famous Floyd V. Filson of McCormick Seminary, in Chicago."

"You two now help out at Village Church, Arcadia, California, don't you?"

"Yes, we do. I am Parish Associate Pastor at Village Church, just as I was at the Lakewood Church, but the financial arrangement is quite different. Instead of a half-time salary I offered to serve at Village Church for the grand total of one dollar a year. The church happily agreed to my terms. The second year they generously doubled my salary to two dollars a year.

"Kirby and I visit older people in the church. I preach occasionally and sometimes teach a Bible class. Kirby is active with the Women's Association and a group called 'Piecemakers.' The Piecemakers group is a craft and needlework group. Each fall they hold a bazaar where they sell the items they make. The funds they raise help to hire a part-time pastor as Minister of Christian Education there.

"Recently, Kirby organized a special program which was a smashing hit. It was a fashion show of various types of wedding dresses. The adult women provided the wedding dresses, and the senior high school girls became models. It was a lot of fun—and it helped to draw adults and young people closer together, as they shared in this joint project."

"*I know both of you have served on several committees and helped with service projects here for the two hundred-plus retirees at Westminister Gardens. What specific things have you done here?*"

"Let me see. I have served as secretary, and as president, of our Residents' Association. In addition to committee work, Kirby now serves as editor of our in-house monthly newsletter, titled *Gleanings*. This is not only for our residents here, but is also mailed out to over three hundred friends. Many of these friends support us by their prayers—and some with helpful gifts."

"*Knowing how busy both of you are, I was surprised to hear you have some health problems. How are you now?*"

"Like most seniors, we have a few problems. Kirby has suffered several bouts with illness plus one bad fall that injured her hip and had her in a wheelchair for a while. I had to have prostate surgery in 1993, but am now all right—thanks to a special medication I receive at the doctor's office once a month."

"*Are there any bothersome side effects from your medication? I know others here who do have bad side effects.*"

"Getting painful shots at the doctor's office is not exactly fun. And I do get hot flashes occasionally, which bothers me—mainly because it sends my wife into gales of laughter every time I tell her I am having a hot flash. She kids me but she has forgiven me for becoming a minister, after she had vowed she would not marry one. And she didn't. I was a naval officer when we married—ministry came later.

"Kirby also kids me because the medicine makes me put on weight. She enjoys ribbing me because I have told her in the past that my trim figure was due to 'right thoughts and clean living.' After all, as the son of missionaries to China, I have an image to live up to."

"*Both of you do so much for others that I fear you may damage your own health from overwork.*"

"That is one side of the service-to-others coin. It is possible to do too much and suffer health problems, but there is another side to the service coin. Serving others can actually benefit our own health. Let me share an example from the great Indian saint, Sundar Singh.

"Once Sundar Singh was crossing a dangerous, snowy mountain pass in freezing weather. He met another man and they struggled on together. Then they saw a third man lying unconscious down a steep slope beside the road.

"'Let's try to go down and help that man,' said Sundar Singh.

"'That would be stupid,' said his fellow traveler. 'We can barely save ourselves. To try to help the fallen man would be suicide,' and he walked on alone.

"Sundar Singh carefully descended the dangerous slope. He managed to get the unconscious man on his shoulders and struggle back up to the road. Soon the unconscious man revived and they kept walking, trying to keep from freezing. About an hour later, they came upon the man who had refused to help. He was dead, frozen to death. The extra exertion of Sundar Singh in saving the fallen man had warmed Sundar Singh's body and helped to keep him alive. He and the fallen man finally made it safely to the next village. The exertion and joy of helping someone had benefitted Sundar Singh himself.

"Serving others can also help us. At age seventy-one, I feel blessed to be able to serve others."

Overcoming Grief While Helping Others

VICKI McCLELLAND JOHNSON

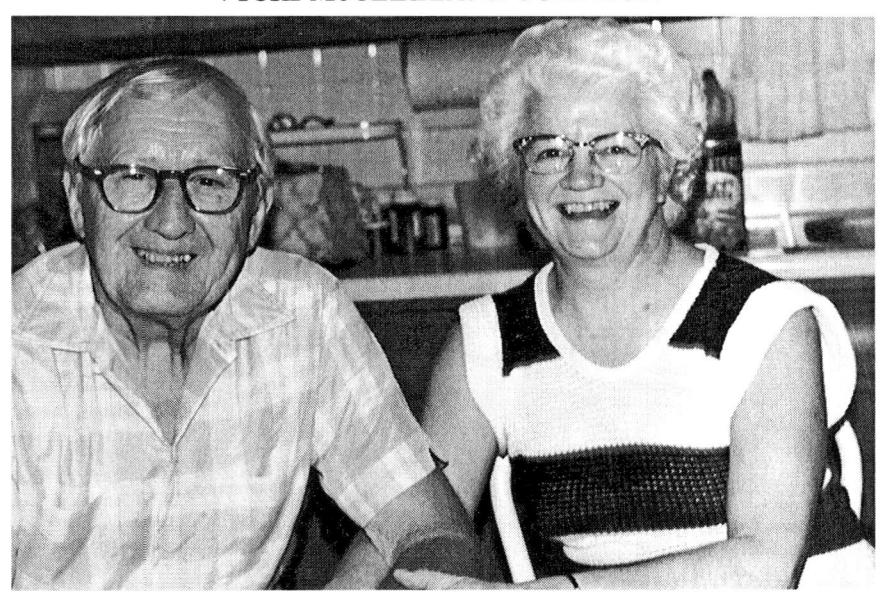

"*Vicki, I have known you since 1973. You were then working at Maryville College in Tennessee, but I don't know what your duties were there.*"

"My duties were many, but my main responsibility was to help in arranging housing, food, and other needs for college students. I was an assistant in the Student Services Office there."

"*As I remember it, you found a late-blooming romance at Maryville College, didn't you?*"

"Oh yes," replied whitehaired, blue-eyed Vicki. "A college dean and long-time friend started dating me after the end of his first marriage. Our friendship rapidly developed into love. The late-blooming romance was all the more wonderful since I had waited so long for it. It didn't matter that I was age forty-four and he was seventy-five. We were both very healthy, active, and eager to start our new life together. I took early retirement at age fifty-two so we could spend more time together. He, Dr. Frank McClelland, and I moved into a lovely new home with a spacious yard and garden."

"*What activities did you have a common interest in?*"

"Many, many things. Even working together in our garden was fun. We raised tomatoes, green beans, corn, etcetera. Sometimes we had enough to share with friends. Our worship, and much of our social life and outreach to our community, centered in our church life. We served on committees, and Frank led some discussion groups. I worked with church women's programs. A few people kidded us about our age difference, but to us it was no big deal.

"After moving into our new home, I decided a good way to get to know our new neighbors was to deliver newspapers to them, and Frank helped me. Later, at the request of a friend, we tried selling Amway products, but after a year of that, we decided that sales was not for us, and we withdrew from that.

"Traveling together was another thing we enjoyed. We especially liked the exotic mountain and ocean scenery of Hawaii, and we found the many pineapple and coconut dishes quite tasty. Frank had spent some time in Hawaii as a marine in World War II; and of course, while on Oahu we visited Pearl Harbor. One day on a bus tour of the island, the bus driver, upon learning Frank had lived in the Scofield Barracks, insisted on taking us on a side trip to the barracks. After thirty-five years, Frank still had nostalgic memories of living there.

"Another exciting trip was to southeast Alaska, where Frank lived with his home missionary parents who were serving at Sitka. It was fascinating to see the yard Frank had played in as a small child, even though the original house had been replaced by another one. Presently, the dean of students at Sheldon Jackson College lives there. We had much to share with each other since Frank had been dean of students at Maryville College."

"*How many years did you and Frank enjoy together?*"

"We had almost twenty-one wonderful years together. Then Frank had a stroke at age ninety-five and lived only two and one-half months after that. Although I hated to give him up, I was grateful to God that in his mercy he did not allow Frank to linger on in a debilitating illness."

"I'm sure losing Frank was hard on you."

"I was devastated! At his age it was not unexpected, but one can never be really prepared when a loved one leaves. It is only by the grace of God that I have been able to keep going, keep busy, and able to meet the public obligations we once met together. I soon discovered that, although friends and family can help, ultimately I had to work my grief out with God."

"When I was in Maryville I saw how great Frank's love for you seemed to be. I also remember a humorous thing he said in my presence, 'I don't mind doing the dishes, but I do wonder why Vicki needs so many pots and pans to do the cooking!'"

"I admire the way you have kept up the volunteer work you have always done. Didn't you help at the local hospital?"

"Yes. I helped to deliver newspapers to patients' rooms. Afterward, we left our unsold papers at the hospital gift shop for them to sell."

"Didn't you also help our mutual friend, Geneva Anderson, as aging and illness disabled her?"

"Yes. I wrote letters for her, paid her bills, and took care of her business in any way I could. I also wrote letters for a blind pastor in a nearby nursing home. And, as you know, I helped to publicize and sell mission story books written by a retired pastor who had served my church in the past."

"What about the telephone helpline work you have done? Since you have suffered pain and loss yourself, I am sure you can sympathize with others who struggle with pain and loss."

"Oh yes. I think my own suffering over the loss of Frank did help me understand and sympathize when hurting people called me on the helpline. Another thing that helped me to counsel them, was that I took the required fifty hours of training to do helpline service. I got a real sense of fulfillment from trying to help others with their problems and pain."

"Have you done any traveling since you lost Frank?"

"Yes, in a limited way. My most interesting trip was to Europe and England in the summer of 1994. That was my first trip outside the U.S.A. It was a wonderful trip, but it was one on which I got lost! That happened in Prague, Czech Republic. I made the mistake of thinking I knew how to get to the designated spot where we were to catch the bus to go to the hotel where we were spending the night. I left the people with whom I was shopping, saying that since I was through shopping, I would go back to the place by bus. When I requested help from police and taxi drivers, they couldn't help me. Apparently they knew the hotel by another name. Finally, after the time to meet the group had passed, I decided to go back to our hotel in a taxi. Thankfully, the taxi driver was familiar with this hotel. I arrived back safely.

"I had learned the hard way that I should have followed the director's instructions never to be out alone! It was a harrowing experience to be lost in a foreign country with no knowledge of the language. But I didn't panic, and I am very grateful, to say the least, that it worked out all right. Now I can laugh about it, but at the time, I was too shook up to see any humor in it."

"How is your health now?"

"Well," said Vicki. "At age sixty-eight, I am blessed with very good health. I walk my pet poodle, Pebbles, every morning and evening (and often in-between). This is not only exercise but enjoyable—it brings back memories of how Frank and I used to walk in the mornings. Both of us took great delight in the beautiful sunrises. I also keep up my yard work, but it is not as much fun as it was when I had Frank doing it with me. Now instead of 'fun' it is 'work.' And I try to eat healthful food and keep a positive attitude toward life."

"Do you have any advice to pass on to others considering retirement?"

"Well, perhaps a little. I advise others to keep not only their physical health and mental capacities strong, but also their spiritual life vital, and hope alive. That is what keeps me going from day to day. I pray each day that God will give me what I need when I need it. I remember his past mercies and know that he is always near. We should all be thankful for our blessings. God has helped me, and I am sure God will help others."

Author's Note:

Soon after sharing her story with me, widowed Vicki met an attractive widower, a nearby church member. She wrote to me saying, "Recently I met Lincoln Johnson, who lost his wife some time ago. We liked each other and 'hit it off' right away." Soon after that, they became engaged, sold their former homes, bought a convenient condominium, and began their new married life together.

Pastoring, Writing, Singing, and Caring for Family

JOE GRAY

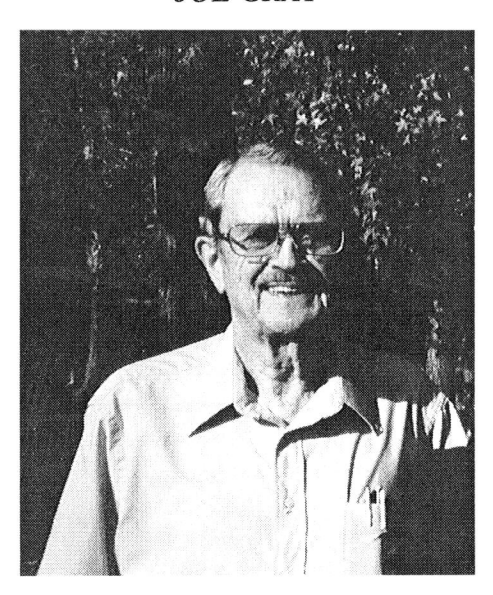

"*Having read your book,* Navajo Sunrise, *Joe, I know that about twenty years of your ministry was with Navajo Indians. What was unique about serving Navajo people?*"

"Well, one unique thing was that my first wife, Mildred, and I lived on the Navajo Reservation. That was almost like living in a foreign country. The customs were different, the language was different, and we were isolated from distant friends and relatives, although we could visit them." Joe continued his story in a voice that was warm and pleasant.

"But what a joy it was to see many Navajo people becoming Christians. I remember one Navajo man who, after much prayer and effort by his Christian daughters, finally overcame his alcoholism. Afterward he began to witness to the power of Jesus Christ to change peoples' lives and bring peace and joy.

"Wanting to serve the Navajo people as long as possible, I stayed on past age sixty-five. But by age sixty-eight I knew I couldn't keep up the strenuous pace much longer. At breakfast one morning I felt 'tuckered out.' My wife said, 'What do you expect when you are awakened at 2 a.m. to take a woman in labor to the hospital? We better retire soon.' Having depended on my wife's wisdom for many years, I agreed. Having worked hard, my wife also needed to retire, and we soon did so."

"Didn't you serve a church as interim pastor after retirement?"

"Yes. I first served a church in Oroville, California. We were to retire to a new duplex in Los Gatos, California, but it wasn't ready when I ended my Navajo ministry in Chinle, Arizona.

"The Oroville Church had been upset by its depressed young pastor who marched up and down the church aisle one Sunday before the service and cursed the people. I was asked to come and conduct a 'healing ministry.' Thankfully, the Church soon recovered its peace and composure. This short ministry helped me realize that I could minister to a non-Indian congregation after not serving such a church for two decades. With much preaching about love and forgiveness, much counseling and prayer, God enabled me to bring healing to that deeply wounded church.

"Our new retirement home at El Sombroso Oaks at Los Gatos was ready for us to move in by the fall of 1973, and we began our new life there."

"Didn't you serve another church pastorate after you moved in?"

"Yes. I was called to serve a small church at Bonny Doon, on a mountain north of Santa Cruz, California. It was an unusual suburb in the forest with a church building that could seat about fifty people.

"Bonny Doon was twenty-eight miles from Los Gatos over curvy highway Number 17. The mountain road was so narrow and winding, with dangerous curves, that I had to drive slowly, taking almost an hour to get there.

"The people became very responsive to my ministry and supported their church well. They had a choir of ten to twelve members. The people also attended worship services on Sunday, and Bible classes Wednesday nights. I was able to baptize two men as a result of the Bible class. When those two husky men knelt to be baptized, many eyes became tearful.

"That congregation had not had any new confessions of faith for many years, but that year the smallest congregation in San Jose Presbytery had the highest evangelistic index."

"What else did you do in those early years of retirement?"

"Well, I decided to study creative writing in a weekly night class. I wanted to write about my two decades as a missionary to Navajo people. In my study I began typing out class assignments and stories from those glorious years with the Navajos.

"The teacher would read to the class what I had written. Then I received many suggestions for improving my writing. Finally, in 1976 my small book, *Navajo Sunrise*, was published. Soon after that the publisher declared bankruptcy but let me have his unsold copies to sell. Thankfully, it was *not my book* that caused him to go bankrupt!

"I eventually wrote four more books, some short stories, and five pamphlets for Navajo Christians. After my eyesight began to weaken, I thought I would write no more but, with my second wife's generous help, I am still at it.

"After my first wife, Mildred, died in 1989, I wrote her biography. I was glad I had saved our courting letters. I titled it *First Things First*. It became a big hit in her small Illinois hometown. It was a valued addition to their local library.

"The last book I wrote was my own autobiography, titled *Stars in His Eyes* (after a friend's comment about me). The most enthusiastic response came from several nieces. One niece in my Gray family, Sue, rewarded me with a gift of a black golf cap with the 'punny' message 'Aging GRAYsfully' written above the brim for all to see. At age ninety-two that is quite a challenge for me."

"Since moving to your present retirement community here at Duarte, California, I know you not only joined the chorus but also sung solos. How did you begin learning to do that?"

"My father sang tenor beautifully. I wanted to imitate the way he sang religious solos in church. He sang so that the listener not only heard good tones but also received a meaningful message, along with the pleasant satisfaction of hearing him.

"Imitating my father's tones, I sang as I walked each day on the grounds of a church near my retirement home in Los Gatos. I also sang as I drove the long miles to and from the Bonny Doon Church I served at that time. As a result the Bonny Doon choir director asked me to sing the opening tenor solos when the choir sang Handel's *Messiah*. I was able to hit the high notes—but I knew I had not become an opera star. I continued trying to improve.

"After the pastorate at Bonny Doon ended, I sang tenor in the choir of the Los Gatos Presbyterian Church. The choir director there taught me to sing from my diaphragm instead of my throat. That helped. I learned to support the tones with what singers call 'a column of air.' Soon I could reach higher notes than before."

"*When did you move from Los Gatos to Duarte?*"

"That was in 1987, and after singing in the Westminster Gardens chorus here—and after singing in choirs for about eighty years—finally I could sing like my dad."

"*What other community service have you done in retirement?*"

"Twice I served as president of the residents' association at the retirement community in Los Gatos. I often showed slides and told about Navajo people's life and customs in surrounding churches and public schools. I tutored four elementary school students who had reading problems. I also did letter writing and banking errands for a disabled friend, and read to her."

"*I have seen some of your art and craftwork. How did you get involved in that?*"

"I like making small things in redwood, which was available in Los Gatos. I made Swedish style Christmas 'trees' out of narrow strips of redwood for family and friends. I also made letter holders. I even made a table and benches for our porch, plus a coffee table and a jewelry cabinet."

"*Knowing the dedicated way you cared for your first wife, Mildred, and your son, David, in their terminal illnesses I admire you as a great caregiver, Joe. What was the most difficult part of that caregiving?*"

"Well, with Mildred's severe asthma, it was difficult to see her wake up at night struggling to breathe. In addition to her regular medication, I learned that massaging her back could help. Many dark nights we struggled together to keep her alive. Finally, the burden on her heart became too great and she died of heart arrest in 1989. I am glad that I could show my love for her by being her caregiver in those last painful days.

"Mildred had helped so much in my ministry to the Navajo people that the Navajo Christians requested that I let them bury her ashes in the yard of the pastor's home beside their church on the reservation. While we were there, Mildred had made our home a hospitality center for all people.

"The most difficult part in my caregiving for my youngest son, David, was the pain of seeing his once healthy body destroyed by the AIDS virus at age fifty-one. I had not even known he was gay until he came to live near us in Los Gatos when he was age thirty-four. I assured him that I loved him and would help in any way I could. The tragedy of his death was doubly hard to face because it came soon after he had finally found happiness as president of the Geneva Players, a drama group producing dramas at Immanuel Presbyterian Church in Los Angeles.

"In treating his AIDS, it was discovered that he was also suffering from 'simple schizophrenia.' This helped me to understand why he had never been able to hold a permanent job, or find happiness in his work until he belatedly studied in a school for actors, and found it enjoyable. He had been an extra financial load during twenty years of my retirement, but I was grateful that I always had enough resources to keep him happy and busy, in spite of his troubles. My love for him never lagged in all those years—and he knew I loved him to the end.

"After my first wife died, God blessed me with a second good wife, Lucy. Now, with me at age ninety-two and Lucy at age eighty-one, we are caregivers for each other. She helps me with my writing and drives our car, which is now impossible with my failing eyesight. We enjoy our life together. Some people thought I was foolish to remarry at age eighty-eight. But marrying a young woman of seventy-seven was one of the smartest things I ever did! Every day I thank God for my blessings."

Retirement: Deceleration or Cold Turkey?

ARTHUR BUSHING

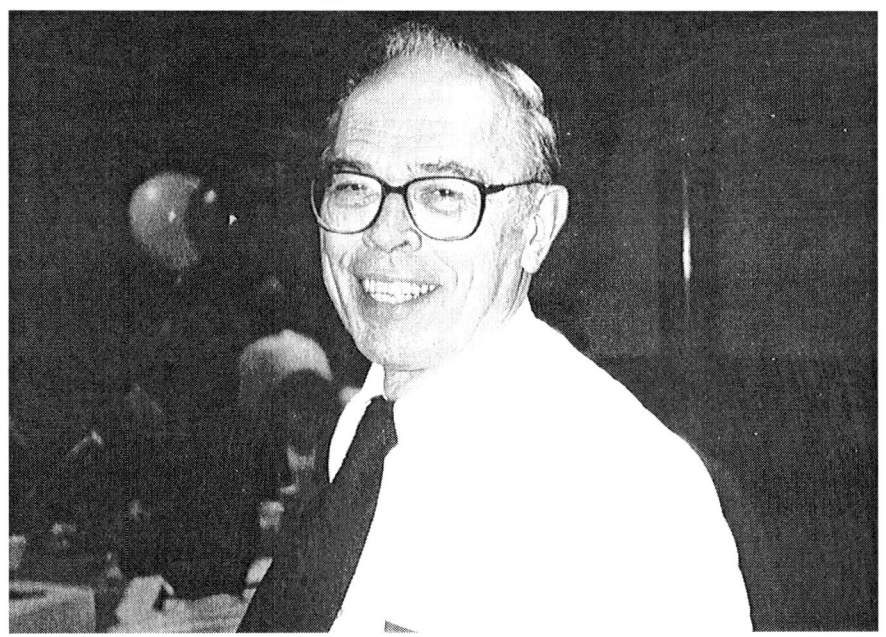

"Art, I first saw you in action teaching English language and literature at Maryville College when I became pastor of your church in Tennessee in 1973. Knowing your talents for teaching, I am not surprised that you continued educational work past the usual retirement age. How have others reacted to your retirement?"

"Let me share with you one reaction I had from a former student ten years before I began to think about retirement. During a visit the man asked, 'What? Are you still here?' He exploded with mock surprise. He went on to recount the pleasures of fishing, hunting, and golfing. The impact of the question was not quite the same as when another student inquired whether I had served in the First or the Second World War. In neither case was the student on the same time clock as mine." A smile brightened Art's face and his eyes twinkled with humor as he told me this. He continued his story.

"Yesterday, I heard a report on retention in the learning process. After six months, we retain little from lectures or even from reading. But from teaching, the report says, we retain ninety percent of the material. I somehow sensed that discovery when I chose teaching as my profession; I craved to learn more."

"At what age did you start making plans for your retirement?"

"I was well past sixty-five when I began to consider seriously the next major change in my activities and then it was with no eager anticipation. The fact is that I have always enjoyed work, was extremely bored in situations of forced idleness in the Army, and could think of no leisure activity that would provide the satisfaction I found in my career.

"In 1956, Dr. Edwin R. Hunter, Dean of Curriculum and Chairman of the Department of English at Maryville College, stepped down from his administration position but continued as department chair and full-time teacher. During the next eleven years, he systematically reduced each area of responsibility, completing his career of half a century at Maryville in 1967.

"For many reasons, Dr. Hunter was my model. He was my teacher, mentor, colleague both in our profession and in our church, and, most of all, he was a very close friend. Dr. Hunter gave me the pattern which I consider ideal for a retirement program."

"When did you start slowing down?"

"Sometime in the early 1980s, I asked to be relieved of some of my administrative duties. At one point, I was director of summer school and of our continuing education program while at the same time teaching almost full time. As chair of the Department of Languages and Literature, I began to look for colleagues who could teach my upper division classes. Although I am again scheduled to teach a summer school class in 1996, I completed my last year on a regular schedule in 1993, the year I became seventy-one and fifty years after I taught my first college class.

"I jokingly taunt former colleagues in response to their questions about retirement. 'Can you imagine life with no committee meetings and no papers to grade?' I asked. I also point out that I can find something to read on the new book table in the library, check it out, and read it. None of that futile dream of saying, 'Well, when I retire I must read this.'"

"Are there things that you miss in retirement?"

"What do I miss? Believe it or not, I miss the fifty-nine steps from the ground to the office I occupied for more than forty years. I miss the interactions with colleagues, staff members, maintenance crew, housekeepers, and especially students. I miss the routine and the daily challenge of teaching.

"More importantly, what have I gained?—more freedom, of course. I have more choices for reading, research, writing. I have been able to pick up projects long-postponed. I can begin spring gardening when the weather permits, not when I have caught up on my paper grading.

"I refuse to use the cliché that I am busier than I was before retirement—in fact, I avoid using the term 'retirement.' I admit, however, that without the pressure of routine, I have lost some efficiency. But I have time for a monthly book discussion, a weekly Bible study; I teach a Sunday school class made up of very alert and intelligent adults. I find more time for exercise, gardening, hiking, camping—more time for cultural events."

"You mentioned teaching a Sunday school class. Are there other church activities you take part in? When I was your pastor from 1973 to 1982, I remember you helped out with many church activities, especially as a leading elder."

"Well, one fruit of my professional slowdown has been the opportunity in my church to join a dozen others at Highland Presbyterian Church who are committed to reading the Bible slowly and carefully from beginning to end. After almost three years, we have just completed the Acts of the Apostles.

"The reading and discussion with this small group has given me new insights into the Jewish faith as a background for Christianity, a greater appreciation for the immense body of truths found in the Bible, and a new understanding of the developing concept of Divinity from Genesis to the revelation of God's nature in the person of Jesus Christ. More than ever, I realize the importance of continuing study, discussion, meditation, and prayer for the serious Christian who seeks to grow in faith."

"How is your health, and your wife's health, in retirement?"

"My wife, Dorothy, and I have thus far had no serious health problems. She has reduced her teaching load of piano students but has not given up that particular love. She is more creative than ever. While enjoying many things together, we have each been able to continue our individual interests."

"*What advice would you give to a friend nearing retirement?*"

"I am young enough that I still ask on occasion for advice. I'm old enough to know that I may not take the advice I receive. What would I say to others regarding retirement? Rather than offering advice, let me summarize a few things I have learned.

"One. Since I enjoyed what I had been doing, I reduced my workload very slowly. Some must end a career cold turkey, which must be very difficult; for me the transition has been smooth. Deceleration has merit.

"Two. No matter how much I have enjoyed my career, it is important that I have other interests I can pursue. I still find opportunities to do some teaching; I can continue such pleasures as walking, camping, gardening, reading. I can attend more cultural events, give more attention to the needs of others.

"Three. My contacts with young people have always been challenging and invigorating. Those contacts will be less frequent, but I have developed friendships across the spectrum of age. The old as well as the young have much to teach us.

"Four. I push myself to exercise mind, body, and spirit. Lethargy, languor, apathy: these are besetting threats as our body slows.

"Five. I have increased the joy of living with more time for keeping up with my geographically extended family, reviving contacts with old friends, developing new friendships, having more time for church-related activities, and finding more opportunities to serve others.

"Six. Mutability is a great theme in literature and a common experience in life. I believe that a mark of one's maturity is the ability to distinguish between that which is mutable and that which is permanent. Each stage of life offers the excitement of the unexpected. Although not all is right with the world, God is still in his heaven. To borrow from Shakespeare's Edgar in *King Lear*, 'ripeness is all' or in Hamlet's expression of the same thought, 'the readiness is all.'"

Planting a "Rose" in Westminster Gardens

BOB McINTIRE AND GAYLE BEANLAND

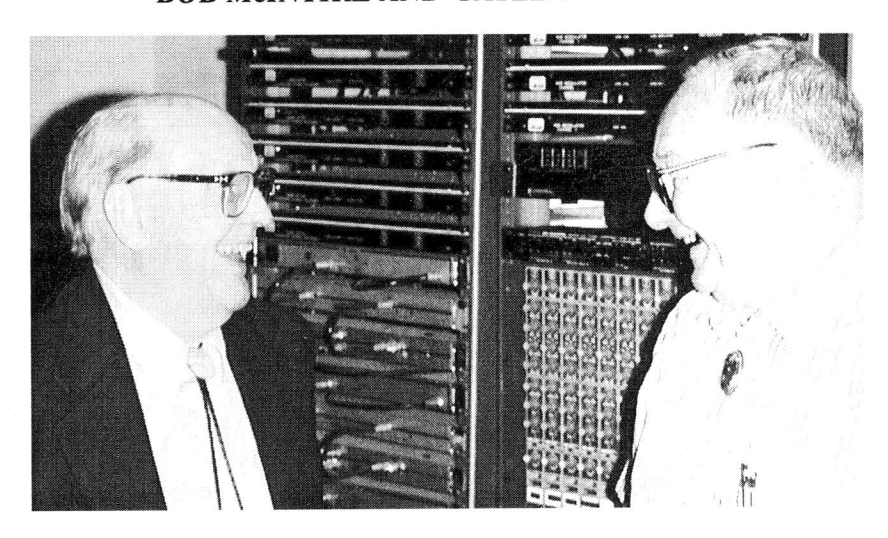

"Bob, before you retired here in Duarte, California, and helped to start our closed-circuit TV Program at Westminster Gardens, I understand you had already performed an audiovisual miracle in Brazil."

"Well, I can't say the development of the 'Centro Audiovisual Evangelico (CAVE)' program in Brazil was a miracle, but it did seem miraculous when, after a long, hard search for a location, a Brazilian farmer felt led to give ten acres of land for that Christian Broadcasting Station. And my experience there did help to inspire me to want to see a closed-circuit TV system here." Octogenarian Bob's deep bass voice was strong and cheerful, as he continued.

"Thankfully, I had help. Francis Sauer retired here after using his engineering skills to help the United Mission to Nepal, and his electrical skills helped a lot. And Spencer England, another retiree here who had used audiovisuals to educate and inspire the young people in the summer camps he managed, was also a great help, especially with his fund-raising skills. Someone jokingly called us the 'human trinity' that got our TV network started.

"But now it is a fourth person, Gayle Beanland, who directs the entire video network for us. Before retiring here, Gayle was director of an audiovisual center in Cameroon and later became a communication consultant to the All-Africa Conference. Gayle has more training and experience in video production work than anyone else here."

"*Yes. When I finish my interview with you, I will go and interview Gayle about his vital part in our Video Production system. How was the original 'dream' for our program born?*"

"Surprisingly, the dream first started when Francis, Spencer, and I began 4:15 a.m. walks together here on our Westminster Gardens grounds. One morning a wild raccoon joined us in our walk, following respectfully behind. But I can't say the raccoon deserves any credit for getting the dream going. I would call the raccoon a 'silent partner' [laughs].

"One morning one of us said, 'Wouldn't it be good to have an electronic bulletin board on TV to announce programs and events for our retirement community.' 'Yes,' said another. 'If we had a closed-circuit TV program, we could even broadcast our various activities so people in our Health Center (Nursing Home) could share in them simply by watching on TV.' As the Bible says, 'old men will dream dreams.' Francis, Spencer, and I are now all octogenarians. And our 'dream' began only seven years ago.

"When other retirees were asked about it most were enthusiastically for it. But some felt it was impossible to raise funds for it, and a few were not sure it was the 'right thing to do.' No one could imagine then that we could develop the great Channel 3 and cable TV programs we have now."

"*How did you get the necessary funds?*"

"Much credit is due to many people but especially to Spencer England, the 'magic fundraiser.' Beginning with small individual gifts from many donors, we eventually raised about one hundred thousand dollars for the project. About half of that came from a generous gift from the House of Rest Foundation in Pasadena."

"*Did you consult with nearby TV specialists?*"

"We got expert advice from a specialist at Azusa Pacific University and from Monrovia Cable TV. And through a friend we got the equipment at wholesale prices. One resident, Forrest Travaille, loaned us his camcorder and Bob Davis, a trustee board member, contributed his own camcorder.

"It was indeed like a miracle when we finally went on the air with a program of daily devotions during Easter Holy Week in 1990. John Shackleford was our first cameraman. The cable TV programs followed later. And now I can reduce my schedule with Gayle in charge of things."

Having finished my interview with Bob, I later consulted with Gayle Beanland about his role as director of our present TV network. To Gayle I said, "*As present director of our video production committee, you know more about the practical and technical side of the system than anyone. Give us your insider's view of what is involved in our closed-circuit and cable TV network.*"

"Well, a lot of effort has gone into planting this 'rose' in our Gardens." Having demonstrated his poetic talent, Gayle went on to show his engineering skills. He said, "Outside of Packard hall, two large TV satellite dishes are located. On the roof of the hall, are assembled two professional TV antennas. A control room is provided in Packard Hall into which are fed the cables from the antennas and satellite dishes. Three banks of electronic controls access the satellites, unscramble the signals, and then distribute TV signals through the cable system. A computer maintains the regular flow of schedules, a video library, and a CD library."

"*How many TV channels are provided?*"

"There is a choice of twenty-one channels, including five national networks with a Spanish language feed; two excellent public broadcasting stations; three independent stations; one international station featuring Arabic, French, German, Indian, and the oriental languages of Chinese, Japanese, and Korean. Satellite feeds include two religious stations, one of which is Faith and Values network financed partially by the Presbyterian Church (U.S.A.) and other denominations; CNN, C-SPAN, Discovery, and Mind Extension University, which provides university courses and technical courses in computer education."

"What other services are provided?"

"To provide a continuous calendar of activities, a computer with a graphic display operates on Channel 3. Featured on the agenda display is a continuous 'crawl' of selected scripture verses. Hal Davis chooses and writes the verses, which are changed every other day. Each morning the agenda for the week is read off-screen, in a 'voice over,' for those having difficulty seeing the TV monitor.

"As background for the Channel 3 electronic bulletin board, a library of excellent music and CDs is maintained and provided by residents. Music from the library is systematically changed with religious selections on weekends to classical and popular music on weekdays, twenty-four hours a day."

"There is a wide variety in the programming, isn't there?"

"Yes. The video production committee provides daily programs in the form of: daily 'Moments for Meditation' provided by selected residents; weekly coverage of the Wednesday Afternoon Fellowship gatherings providing educational and inspirational information; weekly transmission of the worship service from the Health Center; weekly newscasts of worldwide church activities generated from Presbynet and internet using residents as reporters; weekend movies from the Los Angeles County library, and various other sources."

"How do you get qualified helpers?"

"Technicians such as cameramen, switchers, and editors have been trained by the video production committee. We have many volunteer helpers. By God's grace and the help of many friends, this electronic rose is growing in our Gardens. It is providing enjoyment, entertainment, and education needed by the two hundred-plus retirees in this wonderful retirement community we jokingly call the 'servants quarters,' meaning servants of the Lord and his people."

Feeding and Caring for an Angel

HENRY (TIM) LOWE

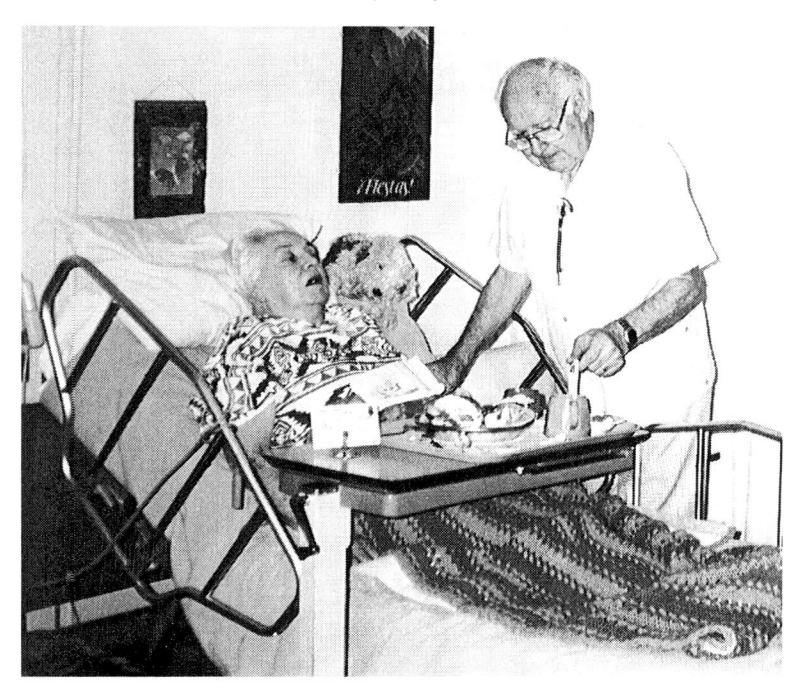

"I'm impressed with your lifelong ministry to people in churches, including one in Campinas, Brazil, and to retired people, Tim. But I'm even more impressed with your present reputation as a 'feeding man.' Why do some people call you a 'feeding man?'"

"Well, I suppose some people call me that because I enjoy feeding God's feathered creatures, the birds. But more importantly because I enjoyed feeding my Alzheimer's wife, Betty. I called that 'feeding an Angel.'" Tim spoke in a deep, warm voice, which indicated love for Betty.

"*First tell me about feeding the birds.*"

"Let me share with you what I did for the birds recently. I put some dry bread crumbs under a cedar tree near my window. First a wobbly black crow picked up a large piece in his bill. He took it to a nearby puddle of water and dunked it in like some people dunk donuts in coffee. He tossed the soggy 'French toast' up a few times then ate it with great gusto. Next a noisy blue jay showed his particular style. He picked up a crumb and hid it in a secret storage place in the cedar tree. Then he rushed back to get more before his other feathered friends could carry away the remaining crumbs. Other colorful birds flew in to share in the feast. I do enjoy feeding these fascinating birds."

"*What was it like feeding your Alzheimer's wife, Betty?*"

"It was like feeding an angel. Let me describe what happened on one typical day. It began with the welcome noise of the food cart being wheeled in from the kitchen. I had already given Betty six kisses: three for her daughters, one for her son, one for me and one for herself.

"To get Betty ready for her meal, the nurse's aide pushed a button and the whirring electric motor raised her bed into a comfortable upright feeding position. Then the aide tied a colorful bib around her neck. Now all was ready for me to feed my Angel. Betty seems aware of what we are doing for her, but she can't communicate.

"I gave her a swallow of water to moisten her mouth, and she coughed softly. Then spoonful by spoonful, I fed her pureed vegetables and meat. Following the prescribed ritual, I gave her a sip of fruit juice, then three small spoonfuls of pureed 'meat,' then two spoonfuls of pureed vegetables. The food didn't look too appetizing to me but she seemed to enjoy it—opening her mouth like a trusting baby bird, to show she was ready for more.

"It is a simple process, but very emotional for me. While feeding my Angel, I recall all the wonderful times we had together as a family. And I thank God for her and for each of our four children, nine grandchildren, and one great grandchild."

"*Recently I saw a photo of you and Betty lovingly touching each tree in a cluster of trees near her sick room. What did that mean?*"

"That is what I call our 'ritual of remembrance.' As Betty's Alzheimer's disease progressed, she lost most of her skills, including the ability to communicate. That's when we started this 'ritual of remembrance.' It became very meaningful to me and I believe to her also. I explained it to relatives and friends as follows:

"Before Betty became confined to her bed, we would often go for refreshing outings, by foot or later by wheelchair, around the beautiful campus of our retirement center here in Duarte, California. While she was unable to speak, or use her left arm, due to a slight stroke, Betty could outwardly show her delight concerning her deep love for God's world of harmonious beauty.

"On these occasions, she would softly brush her right hand along the green hedges, or tenderly hold a freshly picked rose, or lovingly embrace the trunks of the nearby trees, as we strolled slowly along the pathways and roadsides. The incomparable joy of observing her silent reactions to these precious moments, always gave me, her 'caregiver,' a loving reward that frequently made me weep grateful tears.

"This very glad feeling was most evident as we would pass the tree-lined paths, near the Health Center gardens. Here was an unusual cluster of ten small trees, each growing out of a four-foot circular plot of green grass, reaching toward the sky.

"Almost immediately, upon arrival at this memorable cluster, Betty and I would begin a quiet ritual that always brought fond remembrances of the blessings God has given to us through our nine grandchildren and one great grandchild. Slowly, and with much loving patience, we touched each of the ten tree trunks, holding on, as I softly and gratefully spoke the name of each grandchild and uttered a silent, heartfelt prayer of thanksgiving to God.

"Betty and I would then wend our way back to her room to rest comfortably with precious memories. What great joy and pleasure had come into the hearts of these grandparents! We looked forward to touching the tree trunks again and again: one, two, three, four, five, six, seven, eight, nine, ten—until that day on January 19, 1996 when Betty was called to her heavenly home."

Serving Navajos, Hawaiians, Alaskans, and Yavapai-Apaches

JIM DOUTHITT

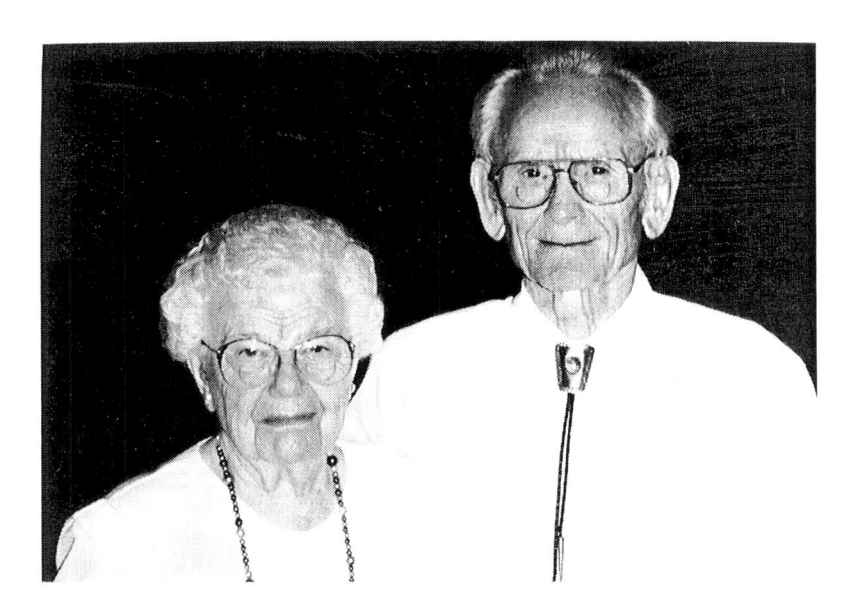

"Jim, I understand you have worked with Navajos, Hawaiians, Alaskans, and Yavapai-Apache Indians. How did you manage to find such exotic and varied places to work?"

"Well, it was a combination of 'Where he leads me I will follow' and 'God helps those who help themselves.' For example, let me relate how my wife, Levia, and I got to serve two summers in Hawaii, after we had retired. It was a matter of cause and effect, which occurred all through our ministry." At age eighty-seven, Jim's voice was strong, his attitude cheerful and friendly.

"Our son-in-law was born in Hawaii, where his father was a pastor for the United Church of Christ there. He knew of a church there that used pastors from the mainland for short periods rather than calling a full-time pastor. The church leader who made these arrangements was a Japanese man, Jack Nishimoto, married to a Hawaiian woman. I wrote him and discovered he had a waiting list, but would add my name to it.

"Then in 1974 the pastor who was scheduled to go there was unable to go, and suggested to Jack that he ask me to come. Arriving there I discovered I had a congregation of three H's: Hawaiians, haoles (people who are not native Hawaiians), and hippies. Thankfully, love for God and one another kept them together.

"I provided Bibles which could be purchased or received free, if unable to buy one. One day I saw a hippie reading one of those Bibles as he sat by the side of the road. He would interrupt his reading to try to thumb a ride from a passing car, then read again until another car came by. I was pleased that he chose to read the Bible instead of some less worthy book.

"Another interesting experience there was the opportunity to bring that Hawaiian church up to date. Their official papers still listed them as a Congregational Church in the *Territory* of Hawaii. I led them to update it to a United Church of Christ in the *State* of Hawaii. Then during my summer there in 1976, I worked myself out of a job by persuading them to finally call a full-time pastor, to this church in the town of Hanalei on the Island of Kauai."

"*How did you get to preach in Alaska?*"

"Another cause-and-effect matter. My cousin teaches marine biology at the University of Alaska in Fairbanks. Knowing I had some building skills, he invited me to come to Fairbanks and help him build a log house that would withstand the sixty degree below zero, freezing, winter days there. We built the house with sixteen inches of insulation in the walls and windows with triple panes.

"While there I was invited to preach at the College Presbyterian Church in Fairbanks, and also at Barrow. At Barrow, the northernmost town in North America, I preached to a congregation of primarily Eskimo and Alaskan Indian members. Also at Barrow I visited the hospital (Presbyterian then, public now) where Will Rogers and Wiley Post were brought after their fatal plane crash."

"*I understand there was quite a contrast between your pre-retirement ministry to Navajo Indians and your retirement ministry to forty families on a small Yavapai-Apache reservation in Arizona.*"

"Contrast is almost too mild a word for the big difference in my ministry to the Navajos and to the tiny Yavapai-Apache reservation, which was about two square miles in size," replied Jim. "My Navajo parish covered three thousand square miles, on a reservation as large as West Virginia—home to two-hundred fifty thousand Navajos. There I was pastor of the church, hospital chaplain, released-time christian educator in seven government and public schools, and field evangelist in thousands of Navajo hogans, during nine years of work with the Navajo.

"I used audiovisual aids with a battery-powered projector, and fifty windup phonographs, which groups could borrow. At Christmastime we had what we called 'Camp Christmas.' About two thousand Navajos attended, some returning home from as far away as Los Angeles. We met on the large Ganado Campus, with a Christmas message to the group in front of the church; then we directed them to the gym where [they received] a bag of gifts, each containing treats and an article of clothing. To feed the huge crowd, we cooked mutton stew in large fifty-gallon metal drums. I will never forget the joy, the close fellowship, and the laughter and fun we shared together there.

"My ministry tended to go in cycles. One of the most interesting cycles was the following. One year the Board of National Missions met at Ganado, and the Directors of New Church Developments invited me and my wife to come to Southern California to organize Mount Olive Church in Whittier. Our thirty-six thousand visits in twelve thousand homes resulted in the church growing to eight hundred six members in our nineteen years there. We took our young people on a 'work camp' to repair and remodel a small thirty-seat church on tiny Yavapai-Apache Reservation at Clarksdale, Arizona.

"When we retired to Sedona we were asked to serve the twenty members of that same little Indian church. We held meetings in the home of a dedicated lay couple, then started Sunday meetings in an Adventist church building. Later we were able to call an organizing pastor. I presented the petition for chartering the church as the

'Verde Valley Presbyterian Church' and approval was received when the deciding church officials were meeting at Ganado. This completed the cycle: Ganado to new church development to Work Camp to new church development back at Ganado."

"Do you remember receiving help from any special person when you particularly needed help with some difficult issue faced in your long ministry?"

"Oh yes. Many people helped me along the way, but I will never forget the special help I got from a Christian lawyer, Vernon Foster. While at Whittier the infamous 'Proposition 14' threatened to scuttle all the fair housing laws in California. Some real estate people, and other special interests, needed to be *opposed* in this. I took a strong stand for fair housing in a public meeting and Vernon said, 'It may cost me my job, but as a Christian I must stand by you in this. We must maintain fair housing laws.' With Vernon's strong support, risking his career, the majority of our church people joined in and we were able to maintain fair housing laws for California—but we did lose some members.

"Another time Vernon gave me invaluable support was when our Whittier church sponsored a Cuban refugee family. At the last minute, the responsible authorities claimed the mother's papers had been 'lost' and she couldn't come. The father and young son decided to come on, to escape Communist pressure in Cuba. It took Vernon two years to get new papers so the mother could join them here, but he never gave up. Later, that Cuban refugee boy became J.C. Penney's man in charge of Penney's merchandising approach to all African-American and Latino people. It was a real success story, which Vernon helped to make possible."

"Do you remember any interesting experience that occurred when you were working with the Yavapai-Apache Indians?"

"Yes. It happened at Christmastime. My wife, Levia, and I often entertained people in our home. Levia always helped in our ministry. This particular Christmas we asked an exclusive boys school if they had any students who had not been invited out for Christmas dinner. They said they had three Iranian boys whom nobody wanted because of hostility to the West by Ayatollah Khomeini, who had just taken over Iran. We not only invited the Iranian boys, we also invited two Yavapai-Apache girls to help us welcome them. One of the girls had been chosen as 'Miss Yavapai-Apache' and was a very attractive and outgoing girl. It pleased us to see how the boys and girls enjoyed sharing their different customs and ideas, even joking and laughing together.

"But there was one tense moment when one of the boys asked me what I thought of Khomeini. My answer may have seemed a little harsh but I felt I had to be honest. I said, 'I think he is so obsessed with hatred for the U.S. that he is insane.' None of the boys said anything, but I was relieved when one of the boys nodded his head in agreement. All of us made some interesting new friends that day."

"You are known here in our retirement community as 'Mr. Fixit,' Jim. Do you remember any particular thing you did to help someone here?"

"Well, I remember several things, but one I was especially pleased with was what I did for Earl and Grace Fox. I not only made a beautiful oriental-type folding screen for them, I also managed to make a hinged 'sliding board,' which allowed Earl to move from his favorite chair to his motorized wheelchair. Earl couldn't walk and that gave him better mobility for several years."

"Do you still play tennis with ninety-year-old Frank Newman?"

"Oh, yes. Recently Frank and I played on the same side for a doubles match. I figured that, with my age of eighty-seven and his of ninety, we had a combined age of one hundred seventy-seven years on our side!

"Another tennis match I am particularly proud of is the day I managed to set up what I called a 'disciples match.' On one side we had Peter and Andrew and on the other side James and John. Making that happy arrangement was a reward for the daily hassle I go through trying to arrange tennis schedules that will keep all the 'old tennis fogies' active here.

"Incidentally, our son and his wife teach in a Navajo school and through them, we still keep up with events on the Navajo Reservation. Including our retirement work, we have been privileged to work with many different ethnic groups for about sixty-five years."

Accomplishing a Musical "Dream" in Retirement

EARLE HARVEY

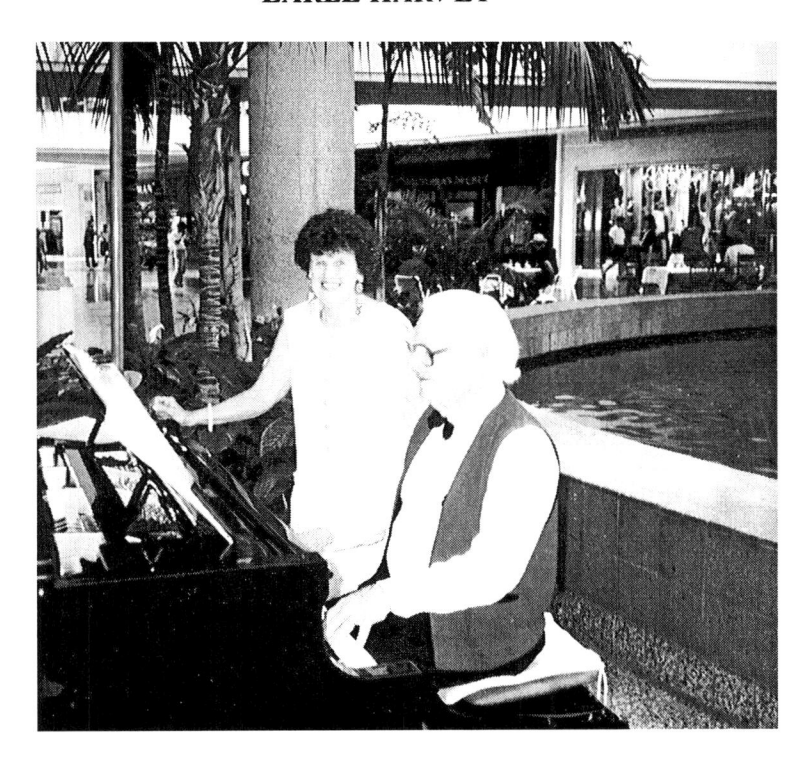

"*I know you and Berneita have had a long career of serving people's needs in many places, since you grew up in the Los Angeles Area, Earle. But now I want you to share what you have done since retiring here in Duarte, California, in 1987.*"

"Well, we had no sooner moved in here at Westminster Gardens and were getting to know you as one of our new neighbors when, as you may remember, you and Lillian invited us over for an evening of fellowship together. You had invited Ken and Sue Carmichael to join us, and we had a wonderful evening getting to know each other. As we talked with the Carmichaels that evening, they asked if we would be interested in some part-time work at their church in West Covina, where they had been attending and doing some volunteer work since retiring at Westminster Gardens. We said yes, and within days I had an interview with the pastor of the West Covina Community Presbyterian Church." Earle's face brightened with a smile as he continued.

"That church hired me to be their part-time pastor of visitation beginning November 1, 1987. Then for three years I visited sick and shut-in people, did a lot of counseling with those who came to me with problems, and even preached occasionally. Amazingly, one of the main strengths of our ministry there was with young couples! As they united with the church, they also became a part of our extended family. They helped us to build a bridge between young and old people there. Some have now moved out of state but, thankfully, have found new church homes where they now live. It was a wonderful experience for me, and for my wife, Berneita, who supported and helped me in all that I did.

"In the first month of our retirement at Westminster Gardens, Berneita and I made plans to travel back to Alaska. Fifteen years ago, in the summer of 1972, while serving as pastor of two parishes in Wyoming, I had taken a group of high school students to Yakutat, Alaska and we helped to lay the foundation of a new Presbyterian church for the fishing village of Yakutat. It was dedicated in November of 1972. The experience of going to Alaska was so wonderful that I promised Berneita that I would take her to revisit Yakutat when we had retired in California.

"Then in October of 1987, we took a month's trip to Yakutat. We traveled by ferry from Seattle to Juneau, Alaska, spent a week in Juneau, flew to Yakutat, and preached for the church congregation there. We then spent a week in Sitka before returning home. It was a marvelous trip."

"Didn't you also serve a church in New Zealand?"

"Yes. In 1992 an opportunity came to go to New Zealand to take over two small churches for a period of four months. A seminary classmate of mine had been hired to care for these two churches for ten months, but found out later that he could stay for only six months. He called me from New Zealand in the fall of 1991 and asked me take over the remaining four months.

"We had four wonderful months of preaching, visiting, counseling, and [experiencing] Christian fellowship there. We began in February and served the two churches of Akaroa and Little River in South Island through May of 1992. Berneita helped those two churches to really 'come alive,' supporting me with her special gift in recognizing people's strengths and gifts and encouraging them to use and share them with others. We still keep in contact with those dear friends in New Zealand."

"What was the next place of church work in retirement?"

"Well, in 1993 another opportunity came our way when we were asked to take a little church in a small lumber town called Glendale, in Oregon. We ministered there for three months. Again we preached, visited, counseled, and did our best to share our faith and love with the people. But it took a heavy toll on Berneita. She came down with a painful rare disease called 'polymyalgia rheumatica.' With that disease, every muscle in her body aches with pain, and it takes years to get over it. With heavy medication, Berneita has improved, but it is still an uphill climb. With her usual cheery smile, she insists she's 'going to make it!'"

"What about your music ministry, Earle? I know that is one of your favorite retirement ministries. And, as your duplex neighbors, Lillian and I have enjoyed free concerts as you practice your amazing piano skills."

"Well, about five years ago, I pursued a 'dream' that I had—which was to play the piano for entertainment purposes at some place where people mingled, such as on a cruise ship or in a shopping mall. My opportunity came when I was at the Santa Anita Fashion Park Mall one day looking at their sand castles display and heard someone playing the grand piano nearby. In inquiring about the matter, I met the person that hires musicians. He interviewed me and hired me! I began playing three-hour sessions at that Arcadia mall."

"After hearing you play, does anyone ever come up to you and say 'thank you?'"

"Oh, yes. One lady came up to me and said, 'Thank you for playing that. It was played at my wedding fifty years ago.' Another time a man said, 'How old are you?' When I said I was seventy-six, he exclaimed, 'You can't be that old; you play too well to be seventy-six!' About a week ago a young woman came up to the piano and said, 'Would you play at my wedding?' 'When is it?' I said. 'In August,' she replied. Then I agreed to play for her wedding. Recently my granddaughter, Tiffany, made my day by saying, 'Grandpa, I want a tape of your playing at the mall for my birthday present.'"

"*What other traveling have you done in retirement, in addition to Alaska?*"

"In 1988 we had the rare opportunity of flying to Finland to participate in a wedding of a Finnish couple. The bride had been an exchange student who lived with us for a year in Waterloo, Iowa. I was glad I had agreed to conduct her wedding ceremony. It was a joy to do so and meet new Finnish friends. After the wedding we visited Copenhagen, Vienna, Geneva, and Paris. It was great!

"In 1991 we took an exciting trip by train from Mexicali through the Copper Canyon of Mexico. And in the summer of that same year we took a Mexican cruise trip aboard 'The Empress,' visiting five Mexican ports: Mazatland, Puerto Vallerta, Manzavillo, Ixpata, and Acapulco. We came back loaded down with exotic photos, exquisite Mexican gifts for family and friends, and enough souvenir memories to last a lifetime. We also travel extensively in the U.S.A., visiting family and friends."

"*What is one of the happiest experiences you have had in retirement?*"

"That would have to be our fiftieth wedding anniversary [smiling as the happy memories came back to him]. It was absolutely amazing how everything fell into place. Some five hundred invitations were sent out. The West Covina Presbyterian Church people took over the responsibility of putting on a marvelous reception and dinner for over three hundred people. The meal was served picnic style in the beautiful park area of Westminster Gardens and other festivities [were] held in the spacious Parkard Hall of the Gardens. The magic date was June 17, 1995.

"All of our six children and fifteen grandchildren attended, along with hundreds of people whom we served and knew through the years, even from our missionary days in China and India. When a wayward celebration balloon set off the fire alarm system in Packard Hall, someone joked, 'See, this is a five-alarm wedding celebration!' And to enjoy it all were more people from the twelve churches we served in California, Wyoming, and Iowa. It was a tremendous shindig celebrating fifty happy years of our married life plus the joyful reunion with many of the people we knew and loved over a span of fifty years. I can't wait to celebrate our sixtieth anniversary!"

"Have you had any unhappy experiences in retirement?

"Oh, yes. In addition to the usual illnesses, disappointments, and frustrations many people face, we had a dangerous car accident. In June of 1992 we took off for Wyoming to visit our children living in the Rocky Mountain areas of Wyoming and Colorado. While going through Yellowstone Park we lost control of the car and rolled over off the highway and had to be taken by ambulance to Bozeman, Montana. Thankfully, we were not seriously hurt, but the poor car was smashed up badly, a total loss. If we had not been wearing our seatbelts, I shudder to think what might have happened."

"How has your health been in retirement?"

"I have had some health problems since 1981. I had prostate surgery in 1981, and I was found to have partial blockage of sixty percent of two main arteries in my heart in 1984. In April of 1994, while attending my brother's stepson's wedding in Susanville, California, I collapsed at the ceremony. My heart stopped. I had to be revived by a doctor and was flown by helicopter to Redding, California. There they did quadruple bypass surgery on me to save my life. I'm thankful to be here today! Later, I apologized for creating so much excitement at the couple's wedding.

"Now at age seventy-six I have arthritis in my lower back, with some pain; defective hearing in both ears; continuing heart trouble since my heart surgery, for which I need constant supervision; plus weakening eyesight from macular degeneration. I tire easily, sleep late, take afternoon rests, and have to curtail activities at times. I have slight bouts of discouragement, but my faith sustains me. And my wife by my side is a real source of comfort and encouragement. I am most grateful.

"Looking back after more than fifty years of a meaningful and joyful ministry, I feel I have been blessed in many ways, especially with a sense of Divine purpose. My heart is at peace and I have a genuine sense of fulfillment. God has guided and used me in his service, throughout each step of life's journey. God gave me my beloved, supportive, wife Berneita, six wonderful children, and fifteen marvelous grandchildren. During missionary service in China and India, and service in twelve responsive churches, God helped me to touch many, many lives for Christ. Every day I thank God for that, and for the gift of each new day God still grants to me."

Taking Widows and Widowers Out to Lunch

FRANK JAMISON

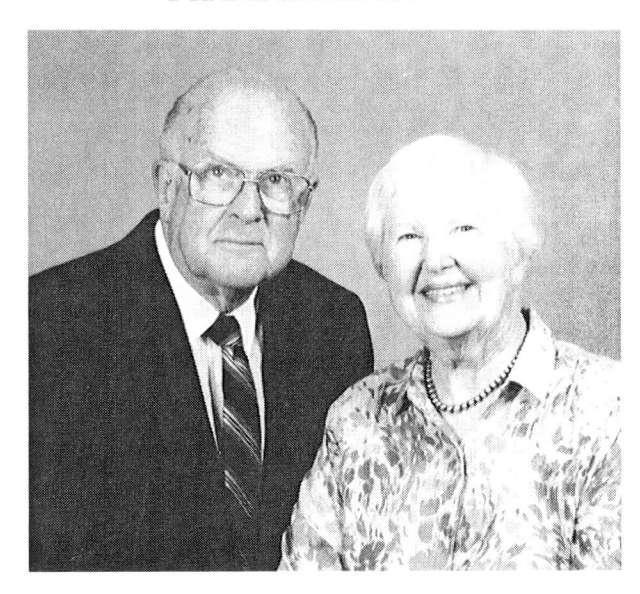

"*How do you feel about being born on income tax day, April fifteenth?*"

"It is a little 'taxing' to put up with the corny jokes I get about it, but it does make my birthday easy to remember. I am now age eighty-three, and my wife, in fifty-three years together, has never forgotten my birthday. In fact, Eleanor is a good wife in every way. Giving me tax exemptions through our three children is just an added blessing. We enjoy our children and grandchildren."

"*What did you do before you retired?*"

"I worked for a statewide bank. I was responsible for supervising loans. I had to approve, or not approve, loans submitted by junior officers. I enjoyed granting helpful loans to people, but my bank had a mandatory retirement requirement at age sixty-five. That came for me in 1978, eighteen years ago."

"Did you make any specific plans for retirement activities before retiring?"

"Not really," responded Frank, smiling and shifting his tall, husky frame in the creaky chair I had provided. "I did what I always do when faced with an important decision. I prayed. Then, after three days of sitting idly with a cup of coffee and the morning newspaper, I got an answer to my prayer: 'Go to your Arcadia [California] church and volunteer to do whatever they suggest.' I did so.

"My volunteering came at a good time for the church. The church leaders had just launched a project to survey all of our twenty-five hundred members to find out how many fell into various age brackets. That kept me busy every day for quite a while."

"What other volunteer activities do you do for your church?"

"I belong to an organized volunteer group called the 'Les Bon Oeufs' (The Good Eggs). We acquired that name because we got the idea to do volunteer work for our church at a breakfast fellowship meeting at a French restaurant, where they served 'good eggs.'

"We work as a group to take people to the doctor or dentist, to paint Sunday school rooms when needed, and to help direct parking when our church has a special meeting requiring that. If one of us is asked to take a sick person to the doctor and we can't do it, we simply call other friends in our volunteer group until we find someone to take our place.

"Our big function of the year, at Christmastime, is honoring our retired church members now living at Westminster Gardens. All of them are former missionaries or church workers. Usually fifty to sixty attend. We serve coffee, cake, tea, and provide some sort of musical program. Each guest receives a gift, such as a potted plant or stationary and stamps. We like to recognize their years of service to the Lord and to people around the world."

"I know you take my single friend, Millie Brown, out to lunch occasionally to provide some caring fellowship for her. How did that begin?"

"That grew out of the helpful vision of an anonymous person in our church who volunteered to provide funds to help shut-in widows and widowers, or any single person, by taking them out to lunch. Six of us organized in 1985 under the name 'TTLC' (Taking to Lunch Club) to provide companionship and sympathetic conversation for people age sixty-five plus. We each have a quota of twenty people, taking ten out to lunch each month. That way we bring a little light, warmth, and cheer into the life of about one hundred twenty people."

"How is it working out? I know Millie likes it. She told me she enjoys having some male companionship occasionally."

"It is working very well, but I did have a little problem last week. After I took three people out together one lady said to me afterward, 'Don't ever take me out with those two again. They are such big talkers, I never got to say anything!' Since our chief aim is to give lonely people a chance to talk, next time I will take her out alone or else make sure anyone who joins us is not a compulsive talker.

"I would like to emphasize that our benefactor has supported this program for over ten years. It is hard to measure exact results but from constant 'thank yous,' and written notes of appreciation, I feel we have developed a gratifying service for our single people and for our Lord.

"Each volunteer files a written report every month reporting his, or her, activity. That report is circulated among the church's senior staff to sift out any additional needs requiring attention. To give you an idea of volume, I have been on over nine hundred lunches since volunteering in 1985. Amazingly, my weight remains constant!"

"Since you retired, did you and your wife ever consider selling your home and moving elsewhere?"

"Eleanor and I have considered that. We decided we had several reasons for not selling and moving. First, we have lived in our home for thirty-two years and like it. We also like our church and don't want to seek another one. Also the hassle of finding new doctors, banks, shopping places, and new friends is a bit daunting. But, most of all, we feel it is important to stay near our children. One lives in the Midwest but one is only three miles away, and another is fifteen miles away. And what would we do with our accumulated 'junk treasures?'"

"I'm sure the people you help are glad you didn't move away. What do you do when someone becomes unable to go out to lunch?"

"I had to stop taking Dr. Ralph Stewart up to the nearby mountains to see the plants he loved," said Frank. "As he neared his one hundredth birthday, he couldn't see very well. While eating lunch there, dangerous yellow jackets tried to share our food. They didn't sting us, but several times Dr. Stewart almost ate one, because he couldn't see it on his brown Kentucky Fried Chicken. We had to give up his beloved mountain trips.

"When Paul Price became bedridden, he begged me to bring him a 'beef dip' sandwich—to relieve the monotony of nursing home food. I can still see the joy on his face as he bit into that juicy au jus beef sandwich. To other shut-ins, I brought cheese and crackers, grapes, or apples, but I always feel sad when one of them becomes too old, or weak, to go out to lunch."

"You look strong. What do you do for exercise in retirement?"

"Nineteen years ago, one year before retirement, I took up golf. It is one of the most enjoyable, and most irritating, games possible. Some days I do well and feel great. Other days I flub, flub, flub, and almost lose my religion. But it is good fellowship, and good exercise, since we pull our own carts up and down the golf course hills. We play three times a week, beginning at 6:30 a.m. and ending about 9 a.m. with fellowship, and mutual sympathy, at a nearby coffee shop.

"I also have a list of jobs to do at home—my wife adds plenty more to it. I never lack for exercise."

"How is your health at age eighty-three?"

"Fine! I'm too cranky to get sick. And I guess I must be living right, eating right, and doing okay with the exercise too. Eleanor is an excellent cook, and we enjoy a good balanced meal together once a day. I get my own breakfast and lunch—and I'm getting pretty good at it."

"What advice would you give a friend who is almost ready to retire?"

"My advice would be: 'When you arise in the morning always have a preplanned schedule for the day. In other words, have a purpose and carry it out—a purpose that is meaningful and enjoyable. Make service to others one of your major goals. Above all, keep a good relationship with the Lord and serve his people in your church and community. Then the Lord will direct and help you.' My personal goal is summed up in Matthew 6:33, '. . . seek first God's Kingdom and His righteousness, and all these things [good things] will be given to you. . . .'"

Hospital Chaplain Work in Retirement

PETER VAN LIEROP

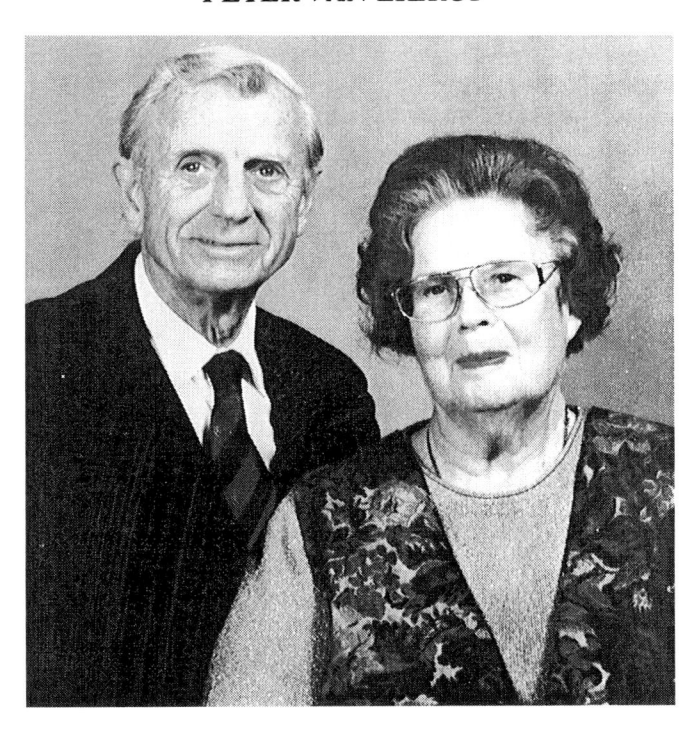

"I first heard of you, Peter, When I visited a mission high school in Andong, Korea, in August 1966. I heard then that you had started that school fourteen years earlier, in 1952. What did you do in Korea after you left Andong?"

"In 1956 I was asked to move to the Korean University of Yonsei in Seoul. I taught religious education, pastoral care, pastoral counseling, and psychology of religion classes there, and for seventeen years, I was the department head for the College of Theology at

Yonsei. The university had only three thousand students when I started there; now it has thirty-five thousand students. In 1977 I retired from Korea to do hospital chaplaincy work in the U.S.A. I needed a change and my wife, Eleanor, needed rest from her demanding work of rescuing Korean prostitutes."

"*What hospital did you work in when back in the U.S.A.?*"

"At first, I was a chaplain at Northwestern Memorial Hospital in Chicago, in 1977 and 1978. Then in April of 1979, I accepted a job as the head chaplain at Sheboygan Memorial Medical Center in Sheboygan, Wisconsin. I served there for eight years, until I reached age sixty-nine and needed to have a lighter schedule." Tall Peter towered above me as he spoke in a warm, enthusiastic voice.

"*What specific things did you do as a hospital chaplain at Sheboygan?*"

"Well, I always kept careful records, and my records show that I visited patients about twenty-five thousand times. I had to answer one hundred fourteen emergency calls for a chaplain. There were one hundred eighty-two 'code blue' visits to patients with heart attacks. I had to comfort parents because of losing babies in four 'crib deaths.' I ministered to thirty patients on their deathbeds. I conducted thirty funerals and did all I could to comfort those families.

"Thankfully, there were some happier duties. I conducted one hundred two marriages, and I was able to help three hundred two alcoholics. I found I could help them through the Alcoholics Anonymous (AA) program, especially 'step five,' which is the confession of the wrong things they have done, receiving forgiveness, and then trying to make amends to the people they have wronged or hurt in some way."

"*What were some of the most unusual emergency calls you received?*"

"Well, for one example, twelve of the calls for emergency baptisms were for people who were dying. Two of them were especially sad; they were for babies born with fatal defects. One poor baby was born without a brain. Another baby was born with all of its inner organs outside the body, without any skin to cover the abdomen. Knowing the babies could not live very long, the parents asked me to baptize them. Imagine how painful that experience was for the parents, and how hard it was for me to try to comfort them.

Even when parents have faith, and can rely on comfort from the Lord, it is still hard to face such a tragedy."

"When did you come to this retirement community in Duarte, California? And what retirement work have you done while here?"

"My wife, Eleanor, and I came here in January 1987; we have been here at Westminister Gardens for nine years. We have good retirement housing and we like the atmosphere. It is like a 'family' that cares for all the family members. And 'Gardens' is an appropriate name for this place because we are surrounded with colorful flowers year-round, green grass, and shady trees.

"Regarding retirement work here, I accepted a job as residents' counselor in May 1987. I have helped many people with worries about health problems, financial problems, and other problems, and I continue to do so when I can.

"In December 1989 I accepted a request to be pastor to senior adults at nearby Glenkirk Church in Glendora. It was a paid position requiring that I work twelve hours a week. My records show that by February 1994, when I left that job, I had made six hundred forty-four visits in homes and hospitals to help three hundred eighty-eight people in any way I could. I also conducted twenty-five funerals and four happy weddings."

"Aren't you now doing hospital chaplain work at the large City of Hope National Medical Center here in Duarte?"

"Oh, yes. In July of 1993 I became a part-time Protestant chaplain there. I work fifteen hours a week with a small stipend. As you may know, this hospital specializes in the prevention, treatment, and cure of cancer, and other life-threatening diseases. They do a great deal of innovative research and are experts in patient care. This hospital is one of the few in the whole country that can do bone marrow transplants. I find my work there a tremendous challenge, but also a great joy as I try to help these very sick people—some knowing they don't have long to live."

"Have you and Eleanor managed to do some traveling in spite of your busy retirement schedule?"

"Yes, a little more than you might think. In both 1990 and 1991 we spent six weeks in Kenya, Africa, serving the churches there as a conference speaker and seminar leader, and as a preacher. I spoke and led studies regarding Christian education and counseling.

"In 1994 we went to Hungary for two weeks, and I lectured and taught classes on counseling at the University in Miskolc. Then in 1995 we made a second trip back to Korea to attend the fortieth anniversary celebration of the high school I founded in Andong; and for the eightieth anniversary of the College of Theology at Yonsei University in Seoul, where I served many years as department head. And we have also traveled out of state to visit our children in New York, Minnesota, and Illinois."

"*Do you remember any patients responding to your efforts to help them with their spiritual needs?*"

"Yes. One day in Sheboygan, a tall young man appeared at my hospital office door. Standing there he shouted, 'I need God!' Speaking as calmly as I could I said, 'Come in and sit down. Let's talk about it.' He then said, 'I owe gambling debts of twenty-four thousand dollars and the men I owe are after me. I try to drown my troubles in alcohol, or block them out with drugs, but it doesn't work. No one seems able to help me.'

"We talked for two and a half hours. He felt his life had ended at age thirty-five. With my encouragement, he kept coming back for help. Later he told me that he had kept a loaded gun at home—and planned to kill himself if I didn't succeed in helping him. I listened patiently to him, guided him to verses in the Bible that showed God's love for him, and prayed with him many times. Eventually he accepted Christ as his Lord and Savior and began attending church regularly. Later he came all the way to California to visit us and stayed a week.

"Recently, at the City of Hope Hospital here, a desperate mother asked me to pray for her twenty-two-year-old daughter who was in a coma. I agreed, saying, 'Even in a coma some people can hear our prayers.' I prayed earnestly for her to know about God's love for her, and God's healing power—raising my voice slightly. Amazingly, she responded, looking right into my eyes as I ended the prayer. The nurse standing nearby exclaimed, 'She has been in a coma for five days, and this is her first response!'"

"*In such serious work, is there ever any humorous incident to relieve the pressure?*"

"Oh, yes. One day I really goofed. I said to a patient, 'Isn't it nice to have your mother here visiting you?' The patient laughed and said, 'That is not my mother, that is my *daughter.*' We all laughed, but I could see the daughter was not flattered to be called her mother's mother.

"Sometimes my wife, Eleanor, kids me when I get so wrapped up in trying to help someone that I come home late for dinner. She says, 'Peter, you had rather talk than eat!'"

"How is your health in retirement?"

"Not too bad for age seventy-eight. Back in 1983, I developed a heart problem called 'atrial fibrillation,' but medication keeps it from being a serious problem. Then in 1984, I had a prostate operation for an enlarged prostate gland, but I have had no trouble since then.

"I do try to eat healthful foods—avoiding saturated fats and salty foods—and I exercise regularly. I play tennis (doubles) four times a week and swim at the local YMCA two or three times a week (one-fourth mile each time). I take vitamins, and I enjoy reading and listening to music.

"I advise others to exercise body, mind, and spirit in retirement. Do work you know well, but don't be afraid to try new things. Above all, show love for others, both near and far.

"Regarding my own life, I feel the Lord has blessed me with a rich, full life—and I am grateful."

A Retired Teacher Who Didn't "Retire"

NELLY FINCH

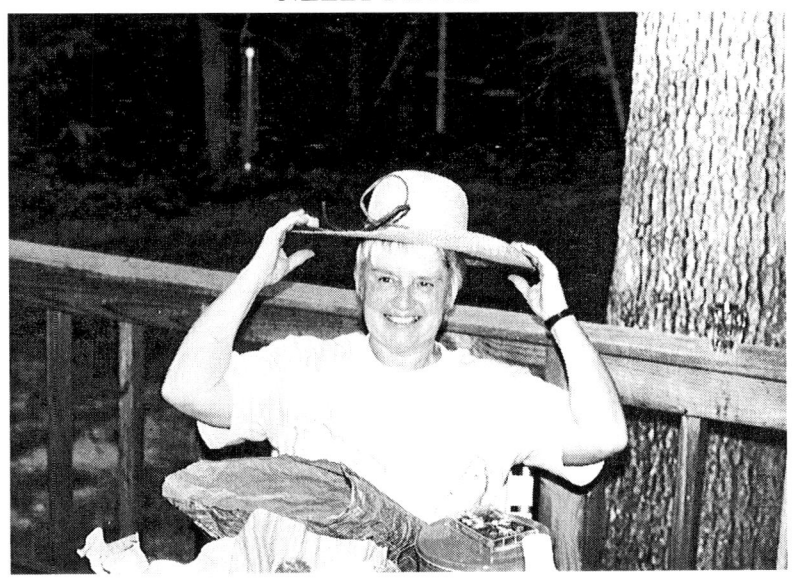

"Since your parents taught me in elementary school, Nelly, I am not surprised that you chose teaching as your profession. How many years did you teach before retiring?"

"Well, it's a little hard to believe, but I taught full time for thirty-three years. Most of those years I taught at Rustburg (Virginia) Middle School. But I also taught eight years at Ely (Nevada).

"Although retired since 1991, I still do part-time teaching. As a benefit of early retirement, I get to work twenty days a year until age sixty-two for the county schools. I am paid double pay. I enjoy this work a lot and don't really feel that I have stopped working. I do some tutoring, help with testing, and do chores like grading papers, running off copies, etcetera (no substituting!)."

"Since you have taken over the family farm in Virginia, after your parents died, that must keep you busy."

"Oh, yes. I take care of cows, chickens, ducks, geese, and guinea fowls. I raise and sell guineas in the summer. Last summer I sold about ninety guineas. I also take care of six dogs (for protection) and twenty-eight cats. All of this keeps me *very* busy."

"*What volunteer work have you done for churches?*"

"I teach a Sunday school class about four times a year. We have different teachers each week. I also participate in 'The Goodtimers,' a senior music group. We sing and play instruments for churches, nursing homes, clubs, and other groups. That is a lot of fun, and I get a sense of fulfillment from doing something to help others."

"*Do you also take part in larger community activities?*"

"Oh, yes. I work at the Campbell County Fair each year. That is not only fun—I get to see a lot of old friends and former students that visit the fair.

"When my part-time teaching job ends soon, I plan to tutor in the Campbell County reading program. There are many students who need help with their reading skills."

"*Have you done any traveling?*"

"I used to do a lot of traveling. I took student groups on trips to England, France, Spain, and Mexico. It was a real challenge trying to learn as much about each country's history, culture, and language as possible during our brief visits. We made some wonderful new friends, and the students found a few pen pals to write to. I also visited the southern provinces of Canada.

"I have crisscrossed the U.S.A. many times, when I was teaching in Nevada. I traveled a different way each time. I also visited the exotic Hawaiian Islands, and the beautiful swimming beaches there. I can still taste the delicious pineapple of Hawaii, but I can't say I enjoy eating 'poi.' It's too 'blah.'"

"*How is your health in retirement?*"

"Well, I have inherited my mother's arthritis, but it isn't too bad, and I intend to stay active.

"I certainly get plenty of exercise taking care of my farm animals, and remodeling our Finch family home. After Mother passed away, and Dad grew older, the house was allowed to go down. The remodeling is almost done and I will soon enjoy a nice, warm, comfortable home. And I can get a 'nice' price if I have to sell it later. I hope that some family member would want to buy it—to keep it in the Finch family.

"Another recent change I have made on the farm is to sell off the hardwood trees (some had begun to die). I replaced them with newly planted pine trees."

"What would you say is your greatest problem in retirement?"

"Probably loneliness. I lost my dad two years ago, when he was age eighty-eight and one-half. It has been hard without him. Thankfully, I have 'cousins by the dozens' and we are all very close; they have helped me a lot. My church friends are also like family, and they help me with their love and support. And my animals help the loneliness, and certainly keep me busy. I have no time to sit around feeling sorry for myself.

"That reminds me, I have agreed to teach in the Campbell County literacy program. Janice Driskill has talked me into giving out programs at the Lynchburg City Fine Arts Center as an RSVP volunteer. And I am also president of our Campbell County retired teachers' organization.

"If I can ever find any time to do more traveling, I hope I can do so with good friends such as those with whom I once spent five weeks traveling together. Our conclusion was that 'any five people who can travel for five weeks in a Volkswagen bus (and share a tent at night) and still speak to each other are pretty good friends.' And two of the campers were children!"

"Do you have any advice to pass on to friends who are considering retirement?"

"I tell them, 'Come on in. The retirement water is fine.' I also advise them to prepare for retirement early—by cultivating interests (and friends) that can carry one through. I also say, 'Retire before many health problems arise. That way you can make a good adjustment to retirement and enjoy this part of your life to the utmost.'

"I have one retired friend who has joined five senior activity and support groups. He needs a great deal of support since he lost his wife to leukemia. He also found it helpful to move to a new location. He needed to get away from the painful memories of his wife, which surrounded him at his former home.

"As for me, with the Lord's help, I'll be able to make it in fine style," said Nelly, always positive and upbeat in her approach to life.

Overcoming a Bad Beginning in Retirement

ROBERT L. CALDWELL

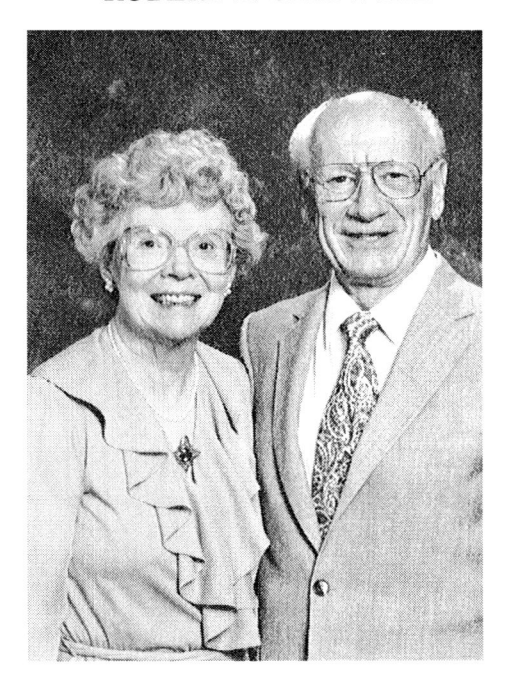

"*Is it true, Bob, that your retirement began badly but then became a good one? You seem happy in retirement here in Duarte, California.*"

"Yes, it is true. After retiring at age sixty (not so old, but apparently too old for a certain midwest church), I moved back to California with some hazy plans for seeking employment in the secular world. After that unhappy pastorate in a church in the Midwest, I felt lost as far as Christian church work was concerned. Was I ever wrong!

"Within three months of my return to California, I was asked to serve as interim pastor of a church in the high desert, at Palmdale. Having never been there, I hesitatingly agreed, and was off to Palmdale and to what I can only call my 'salvation.' The love of the people in that congregation was so strong and so rich that I felt 'found' again by some of God's finest people. After just six months at Palmdale I came back to the 'low country' feeling *high*! And I was eager to serve once more." There was joy in Bob's deep voice and his face glowed as he continued his story.

"Suddenly I was asked to go to a sad little congregation up in the foothills, at Shadow Hills, California. Due to a regrettable problem, responsible leaders in the Presbytery removed both the pastor and elders from their positions of power in that church and sent me into the ring! The people did not ask for me, and no doubt some did not want me, but that noble church put up with me for three and a half years. My first Sunday in that church pulpit, I faced a half-filled church with most of the people sitting there with folded arms and grim faces—daring me to say something wrong (or maybe right).

"I was determined to renew them with one tremendous sermon on the healing 'grace of God.' To my relief, many thanked me for that sermon, and I felt the healing process had begun. Gradually, people shared with me the pain they felt from that divisive strife in their church. We prayed together and even did a little weeping together from the emotional strain on all of us. By God's grace the healing church began to grow and move forward. At the end of my time there, the ruling elders gave me new license plates for my car bearing the Greek word for grace (*xapis*). At the farewell reception, one elder said, 'You have been shoving the grace of God down our throats for more than three years. Now we want you to take it with you!' Thankfully, part of God's grace was my wife, Anna, who helped me to comfort and heal those hurting people.

"I am happy to report that under the guidance of a new and dynamic pastor, the Shadow Hills Church did what every church ought to do. It became a growing church, and today is one of the finest churches in that Presbytery. It is filled with talented people who work for God's glory, developing good programs and an effective outreach to others."

"Didn't you also sell some real estate during that period?"

"Yes. Since I was listed on 'the books' as part-time (and that is a bit of a joke among ministers), the ruling elders gave me permission to do something I had dreamed about for some time, selling real estate. I went to real estate school, became licensed, and sold real estate for four years in Toluca Lake, California. That is a wealthy enclave that includes many TV and movie stars. I tried to sell Walt Disney's former home for three million dollars, but couldn't find a willing buyer with that much money. Of course, I didn't have money of my own to buy that home for my own 'home among the stars.' Work there was fun, not at all diminished by the fact that I was a 'token male' in a real estate office with a staff of fourteen women. Being the only, lonely man among fourteen formidable women, I still didn't have to sue a single one of them for 'sexual harassment.'

"Following Shadow Hills I worked part-time at St. Mark's Presbyterian Church in Van Nuys, California. My wife, Anna, and I developed strong friendships there as members of a group called 'Saints and Sinners.' That social group made church life fun as well as meaningful. Despite my so-called leadership role, I was not necessarily one of the 'Saints.'"

"How did your work in New Zealand come about?"

"Well, our work in New Zealand had its beginning when my wife's college roommate married a New Zealand soldier during World War II. Later he became famous as a brass band leader, performing here in the U.S. as well as elsewhere. He was also a judge in international competitions. They, Norman and Evelyn Goffin, visited us many times. During a visit in 1980 they said firmly, 'We have come to see you many times, and you have never visited us in New Zealand. We are not coming back until you come down for a visit.' With that challenge, the next year Anna and I, accompanied by one daughter and a dear friend, flew south for a delightful experience that we repeated the next year.

"That second year I added my name to the list of American pastors who wanted to serve churches in New Zealand. While waiting, I served a church in Burbank for fourteen months and had a 'second go' at Palmdale for another six months. Then came the word! A large church in Auckland, New Zealand had just 'lost' its pastor. Although it was a temporary loss, they needed a <u>locum</u> (their wonderful word for a temporary fill-in) while their pastor 'itinerated' around the churches and parts of Southeast Asia, as elected head of their national Church.

"What a thrilling experience we had at Somervell Memorial Church in Auckland. Never did six months go past so quickly, and with such joy. Our neighbor across the street was none other than the famous Sir Edmund Hillary who, with his guide, was the first to climb to the top of Mt. Everest. The final night in Auckland, while we were enjoying dinner with one of the church families (one of many new friends developed there), a telephone call came saying, 'next year would you be willing to come to St. Columba's Presbyterian Church in Havelock North?' Anna and I welcomed the opportunity to return to New Zealand.

"We went, and found that we had a church with a <u>session</u> (ruling body) of forty-eight elders and a board of managers (trustees) of twenty-four! And standing room only on Sunday mornings! What a 'high' for a retired, retreaded preacher! There were upwards of fifty children who gathered in front for a children's talk, and when they left for Sunday school, their seats were filled with those who had been standing in the aisles. What a glorious way for a minister who had once been 'lost' because of an unhappy experience in a Midwest church to be 'found' at the end of his career.

"Since serving in New Zealand, we have had many visitors from that beautiful land come to our home here, and we have taken more than one hundred Americans on tour to New Zealand. When they return they say they 'own' a piece of New Zealand—because it will live forever in their minds and hearts.

"After overcoming the pain of that forced termination of my job at age sixty, my retirement has been a very enjoyable and meaningful experience. And my blessings haven't ended yet."

Retirement in Japan, Then in the United States

MILDRED (MILLIE) BROWN

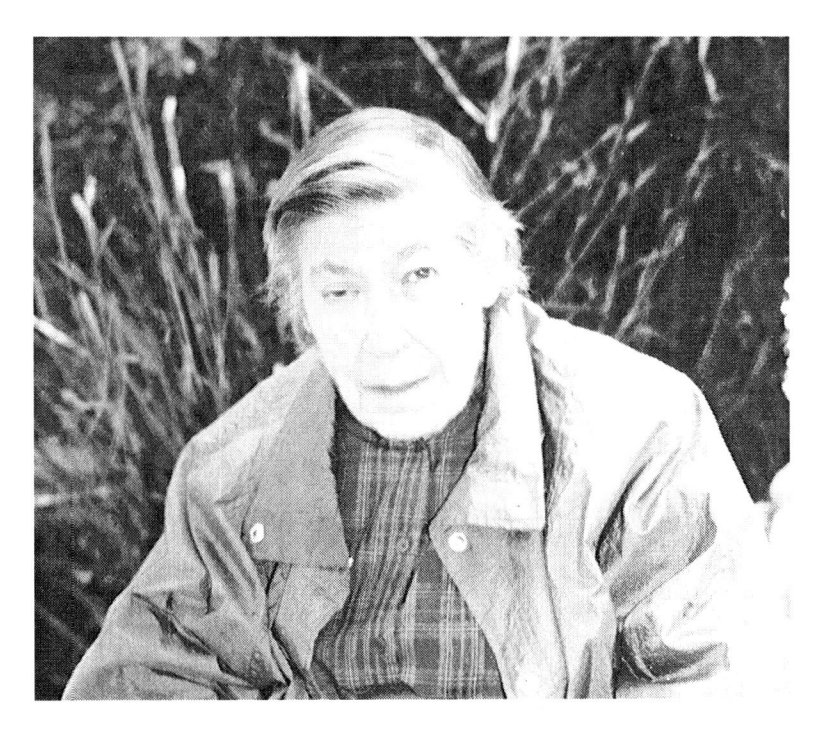

"How long did you serve as a teacher in Japan, Millie?"

"I taught at Hokusei Gakuen (North Star School) in Japan for thirty-four years. It was a happy, beneficial experience, but it did have its ups and downs." A wry smile flitted across Millie's face as she spoke, brightening her wan countenance.

"What was the most difficult experience you had while teaching in Japan?"

"That would have to be the tragic fire at my school in Sapporo in December 1963. That night, part of the school was destroyed, or badly damaged, by fire. The fire started about 8 p.m. in an art room. Quickly it spread to the high school library and destroyed it before anything could be saved. Then it went into the four-year college section, burned off the third floor, and damaged the two lower floors so badly that the whole building ultimately had to be torn down. It left the high school with no chapel, art rooms, cooking rooms, sewing rooms, music rooms, or library. It left the four-year college with no roof over its head. Fortunately, no one was hurt.

"As I stood watching the fire, I was made vividly aware of how much Hokusei meant to the students, alumnae, and friends. My shoulders were wet from the tears of students who stood around me weeping, and I wept with them. I couldn't have taken a picture of the burning building, for I was so emotionally involved that it would have seemed almost sacrilegious. Thankfully, the classes began again in temporary quarters and there was a wonderful spirit among the students and faculty. But I feel pain every time I remember that horrifying experience."

"*Do you remember any especially happy teaching experience in Japan?*"

"Yes. I especially enjoyed the English plays put on by the students during our annual school festival. The students in the English Speaking Society always did those plays well. I think my favorite was the one they did about Helen Keller and her teacher [*The Miracle Worker*]. I was their coach and advisor. That year's performance was outstanding. For one thing, the girls put an incredible number of hours of painstaking work into it, and the work paid off.

"Much of the story was portrayed by action rather than by words, since Helen couldn't talk. And the plot is simple and straightforward. It was a deeply emotional experience for all the participants. The entire cast burst into tears the minute the last curtain dropped. The struggle to enter into the world of the blind and deaf child had become their struggle, and it left them emotionally and physically exhausted. They had selected the play and for those students, it became the greatest learning experience of their junior college life. I will never forget the joy of that experience, myself."

"Didn't you actively retire in Japan before coming to this retirement community in Duarte, California?"

"Yes. In 1982 I reached the mandatory retirement age of sixty-five, but my school offered me the welcome opportunity of staying on five more years under a special arrangement. That meant that I was completely supported by the school rather than by the Presbyterian Church in the U.S.A. I wanted to remain there until 1987, when Hokusei would celebrate its one hundredth anniversary. My five years of retirement in Japan were the best years of my life. I loved every minute of it. To retire in Japan was the best decision I ever made."

"Didn't you have some health problems after you retired in Japan?"

"Yes. In 1986, after four years of retirement in Japan, I noticed some signs of possible breast cancer. There were no 'lumps' in my breast but the nipple in my left breast had turned inward in a very unusual way. I went for a check up. Thankfully, God led me to the number-one breast cancer doctor in Japan, Dr. Asaishi, a doctor I came to respect highly. After careful examinations, he ordered me to enter the Idai Hospital (The Medical Hospital for Sapporo Medical College). After confirming I did have breast cancer, he recommended that I have my left breast removed.

"It was a shock but after much thought and prayer I said to myself, 'At age sixty-nine and still single, I will never need that breast. Why not do the safest thing and let Dr. Asaishi remove it?' And I did so. The doctor put me on the chemotherapy medicine <u>Tamoxifen</u> and that kept me in remission for eight years. In 1994, after seven years of retirement here, the cancer recurred. This time in my bones, with the danger of spreading elsewhere. Now, in 1996, I am on prescribed chemotherapy and have to struggle to keep going."

"Before the cancer recurred, didn't you teach English in several communities near your present retirement home in Duarte?"

"Oh yes. I was asked to teach English to immigrants from Mexico at a nearby social service center called 'El Calvario.' After teaching orderly students in Japan for thirty-four years, it was a challenge to teach young mothers with crying babies in their arms—while older children got into fistfights nearby. That chaos continued for about two years when, to my relief, the center decided to end that rather futile attempt to teach with so many distractions.

"Imagine my surprise when I was asked to teach Japanese students again—here in the U.S.A. They were the Japanese wives of businessmen from Japan who were sent here by their Japanese companies. These young women had children, but they could afford to put them in a kindergarten, nursery, or public school. The six young Japanese wives in my class were eager to study English as a second language and were good students. Teaching them brought back happy memories of teaching in Japan. At first we met at an Arcadia, California, church but later had to meet in my apartment. They often brought food to share, especially when we had a farewell party for one of them when their family had to move back to Japan.

"Only one of them was a committed Christian, but most of them showed genuine interest in the Bible. Three of them picked up a copy of the free New Testaments in Japanese that I left on a table for anyone who wanted a copy. One of them, Setsuko Nomura, had studied the Bible in Japan at Tsuda College in Tokyo. Her teacher had been my missionary friend, Dorothy Havlick.

"Since they were facing new customs and cultural values here in America, I made an effort to help them with any problems or questions they might have about the 'strange' way we Americans think and act. I discussed current events with them, providing duplicated copies of pertinent articles from *Reader's Digest*. We met from one to two hours weekly and I dismissed them in time to pick up their children for lunch.

"One of them laughingly told us about a mistake she and her husband made at the supermarket. They couldn't find the cream for coffee called 'half-and-half.' When the husband saw something called 'buttermilk' he said, 'That must have butter in it like half-and-half. Let's buy that for our coffee.' Imagine the look on their faces when they got home and tasted that buttermilk. They quickly spit it out in the sink.

"One day one of the women came running into my apartment and said, 'You must come quickly and help one of your students. A policeman has caught her!' I rushed out and the policeman said, 'She didn't stop at the traffic stop sign—she just slowed down a bit.' 'Yes, I did stop!' said the excited student. 'Besides, I was late for Miss Brown's class!' (Without realizing it, she had just proved the policeman's point.) The policeman decided not to give her a ticket but did require her to attend a traffic school class."

"Didn't you also do some literacy teaching for older women who couldn't read?"

"Oh, yes. One big black lady named Tempe did very well in those weekly classes at the Duarte Senior Center, lasting about one and a half hours each time. But I never got very far with a very confused white lady named Marcella. She tried but it seemed she just couldn't learn to read—although her husband could read fairly well. The best Marcella managed to do was to proudly announce to me that she had learned to read the sign that said 'Taco Bell.' After four years she gave up on me saying, 'I want you to find me a *good* teacher.' By that time my cancer had recurred and I had to give up teaching anyone. I hated to leave my friend Tempe with no teacher because she was making good progress."

"How long did you edit our retirement community newsletter, The Gleanings?"

"I edited that newsletter for about four years. Katie Turner helped me but I had the major responsibility for getting out over two hundred copies each month. Collecting and sharing the news of our community was fun in a way, but it was a bit of a hassle to meet the deadlines and squeeze too much news into too little space. I could never do that now."

"How is your health now?"

"Not good," responded Millie. "At age seventy-nine, with recurring cancer and side effects from some chemotherapy, I barely manage to keep doing all the things I need to do to just keep going. I have dizzy spells, which make me fall frequently, and I feel tired most of the time. Using a cane and a special walker, I manage to go to the dining hall and do things nearby. But my former two-mile walks to the bank and supermarket are no longer possible. If you try to call me on the telephone, be sure to let it ring seven or eight times—to allow me time to get there. I missed two calls today because they didn't let it ring long enough.

"One thing that brightens my present dark days is reliving the happy experiences of the past. One especially happy event occurred in 1989. I was honored by the Japanese government. I received the Japanese Kunsho Award 'Order of the Sacred Treasure, Gold Rays, Rosette.' It was rewarding to receive this acknowledgement of my contribution to English teaching in Japan, and in trying to promote mutual understanding.

"Another bright memory is my enjoyable five-week visit to the new Hokusei Junior College in Wakkanai, Japan in the summer of 1990. Wakkanai is Japan's northernmost city and cold in winter but pleasant in summer. I felt God led me there not only to rejoice at seeing the new Junior College but also to cheer up a new missionary couple teaching there. They, Barb and Brad Beachy, knew little Japanese and were longing to chat with me in English. It was a wonderful time of fellowship together, and it was a joy to be able to comfort and encourage them as they taught English to Japanese students. It was a lonely, isolated situation, for two new Mennonite missionaries from Goshen College in Indiana. In-between teaching courses in English composition and Bible classes, I enjoyed many happy hours with Barb and Brad—plus informal English conversation with Japanese students.

"And now, in spite of my recurring cancer, I don't want to be pessimistic. God has enabled me to teach in Japan for thirty-four years—and continue teaching here for about five years. Many good friends in Japan and in the U.S. write me, visit me, and pray for me. God has blessed me in the past and continues to bless me today."

Author's Note:

A few months later Millie went to her heavenly home, passing away peacefully, almost as if going to sleep.

Choosing Variety in Work and in Retirement

LEROY (ROY) ENGELHARDT

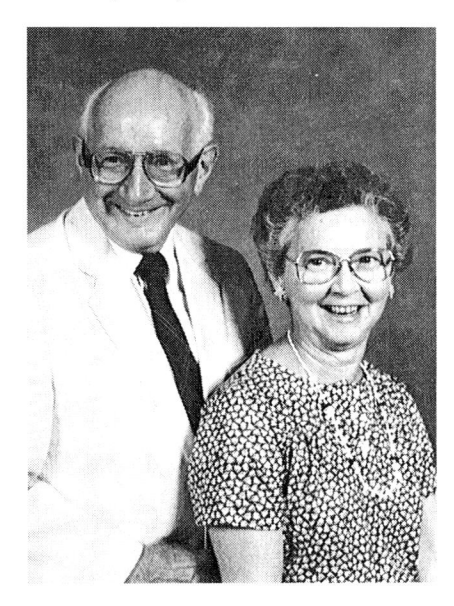

"Before getting into your retirement story please share a bit of what you did before retirement."

"Before retirement, my wife, Mildred, and I worked in places as different as the National Field (where we organized new churches) and the large International Church of Lima, Peru, with many different nationalities and denominations represented. In Lima, Peru, I not only helped with church work but also taught at San Marcus University there. San Marcus is the first university established in the Western Hemisphere—a fact I was surprised to discover. We enjoyed working with new friends there. Thinking back, I realize we have made new friends in many places, some as different as a chatty cab driver in New York City and a quiet shepherd in the high Andes Mountains in Peru.

"I could say the loss of most of my gray hair was due to the stress of moving around so much. But the truth is I enjoyed my varied ministry in many places, and God helped me to overcome whatever stress I met along the way." Flashing his bright, contagious smile, Roy continued.

"The eighteen years prior to retirement, I was a member of the faculty and head librarian at the oldest theological seminary in the country, New Brunswick Theological Seminary in New Jersey. Retiring from there, we moved from the exciting northeastern part of the country, where we were surrounded by a large university, to land we had on the edge of the scenic Great Smoky Mountains in Tennessee."

"*What led you to choose Maryville, Tennessee as your place for retirement?*"

"My wife, Mildred, and I thought carefully about what kind of retirement location we wanted. We wanted a place where we had educational stimulation. Maryville College, where I had taught for seven years at the beginning of my career, and the University of Tennessee in nearby Knoxville offered me free classes.

"I was able to take courses from agriculture (became a 'master gardener') to architecture. The local library had college extension classes in literature, and travel lectures.

"We also wished for good medical facilities and found them here. There were specialists connected with our county hospital, as well as several large hospitals in nearby Knoxville—only fourteen miles away.

"We desired cultural opportunities which came through the college and university offerings. We soon got subscriptions to the opera, plays, and orchestral concerts. We also attended such events as the ethnic Scots/Welsh games. And I had classes in drawing and art appreciation.

"But most of all we sought a good church life for spiritual stimulation. My wife is very active in the women's activities and music at Highland Church. And I have never been so busy in the service of the Kingdom through work on local and area church committees. It has indeed been satisfying for both of us.

"Didn't you also serve several churches in the Maryville area after retirement?"

"Yes, the four churches I served were small but it was a rewarding experience. I sought to help them with beneficial preaching, visiting, and counseling. And they helped me and my wife by becoming cherished friends. After being away from Maryville for thirty years, it was a joyful surprise when someone would come up to me and say, 'Welcome back to Maryville! You were my teacher here many years ago.' That helped to make us feel welcomed and appreciated. Friendship here is more than a chamber of commerce slogan."

"What were the four churches you served in retirement? From 1973 to 1982 I served Highland Church in Maryville, where I understand you and your wife attend now. I may know the churches you served."

"They were Eusebia, Fork Creek, Wilson Station, and Baker's Creek."

"What a coincidence! While in Maryville, I preached and showed slides of our missionary work in Japan at both Eusebia and Baker's Creek churches."

"What is your retirement home like?"

"Our comfortable retirement home is located on about seven acres of land on Wilkinson Pike. We bought an inexpensive manufactured house which suited our purpose to a T. It has one floor, ground level, master bedroom with bath, guest bedroom with bath, study for my books and TV, and large dining and kitchen facilities.

"Our extra large lot has space for a garden, fruit orchard, and a home-designed and built 'Japanese garden.' One of our three children has moved onto this land with us and helps with the maintenance. His family has provided two wonderful grandchildren to enrich our lives."

"I understand you have done quite a bit of traveling since you retired."

"Oh, yes. One of the reasons I retired two years early, at age sixty-three, was to pursue some travel while we were still healthy to enjoy it. We visited Morroco—yes, I rode a camel and visited the Berbers in North Africa—I had a Turkish bath in Istanbul—in a four-hundred-year-old establishment. I sailed on a sailing schooner out of Maine and cruised to Alaska, the Mediterranean area, and the Caribbean.

"I was chaplain on several voyages to scenic places. I sailed around the world with visits to China, India, Oman, and on through the Suez and Panama canals. More recently Mildred and I visited Ireland, Wales, and Scotland. And one of my favorite expeditions led me three times on pilgrimages to the Holy Land. It was a special joy to visit the land where Jesus walked, talked, and then died on the cross to save us. I feel greatly blessed to be able to travel like this."

"I understand that your wife, Mildred, has been very supportive throughout your ministry, in addition to her own music ministry and other work. And I'm sure she also enjoys retirement."

"Well, I must point out that while men retire from their life's work, wives do not. Thus there is a need for her sense of retiring too. For example, having someone to help in the household chores, and going out to restaurants more frequently. My helping to lighten Mildred's household burdens doesn't mean taking over her world, but it does mean sharing her burdens in a helpful way. Thankfully, God gives me the strength, ability, and love to do it.

"For both of us, retirement means taking time to exercise the body, mind, and spirit—and striving to keep our sense of humor in spite of problems that come with aging. At age seventy-five, I am grateful to have a sense of security, adventure, and continuing growth."

Caring for God's Creation: Birds, Animals, and Humans

HELEN FURGERSON

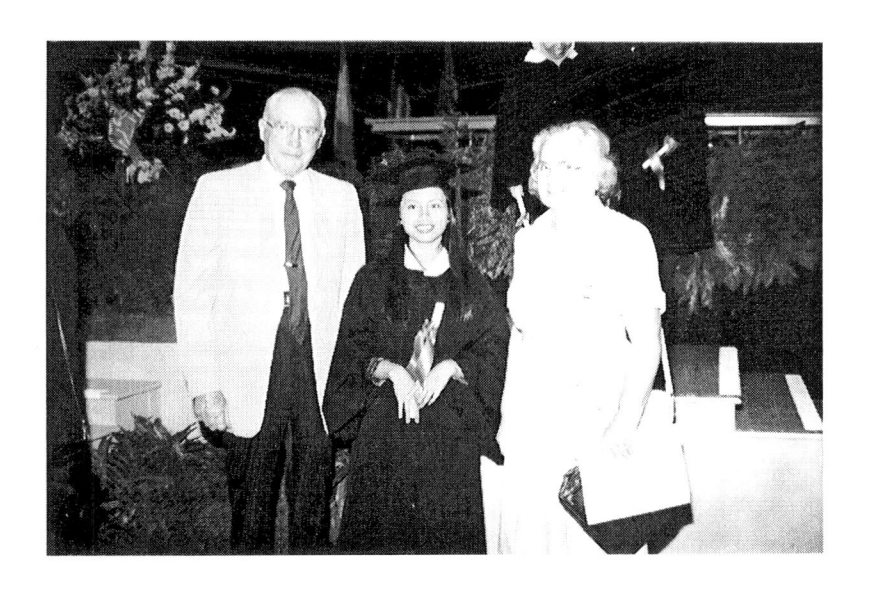

"What did you and your husband do before retirement, Helen?"

"Bill is a professional engineer, and he retired as one of the vice presidents of a company now called 'York International Corporation,' which had about five thousand employees in York, Pennsylvania. I was an unprofessional volunteer who had cooked dinner for Japanese, French, Dubai, and other business friends; written payroll checks for York Symphony Orchestra; fed baby birds; and looked after pets of many kinds.

"One of our favorite pets, and one that retired with us, was a ten-ounce squirrel monkey—given to us as a baby by a friend when we were in Del Mar, California."

"When did you retire to your present home in Tennessee?"

"In the early fall of 1980, we sold our house in York and hit the road for Tennessee. We were both near our sixtieth birthday. Bill had finished his work projects, was physically exhausted, was financially secure, and we did not look forward to spending another cold, long winter in York."

"What is your retirement housing like?"

"Our housing is a three-bedroom, one and a-half bath, two-story home. It is about two thousand square feet in size, and we have a double garage and a greenhouse located on about eighty acres of hills and hollows. This is part of the 'George/Furgerson' family farm in Blount County, Tennessee. Since we built most of the house ourselves, contracting out only part of the work, we know exactly who to blame for the blemishes and warts that appear. In fact we have photographs to prove most of what was done. My maiden name is 'George,' and my brother and I are both here on the 'George/Furgerson' farm."

"How do you spend most of your time in retirement?"

"Well, living in the country provides us with opportunities for work of many *new* kinds. Bill even overhauled and repaired a 1940s-era Ford tractor and then used it to 'bush-hog' the overgrown bushes from our roadsides, orchard, and wherever the land is level enough to use the tractor. We drag out fallen trees for firewood, take grandchildren for a tractor ride to the lake and to pick blackberries.

"We have a garden with both vegetables and flowers. We are slowly learning how to plant in order to receive some benefit in produce in addition to exercise. Last year the tomatoes were great, the habanero peppers were terrific, but wild deer greedily ate up our okra and corn. We have more seed and will try again, finding some way to scare off the beautiful but troublesome deer.

"Bill (officially W.T.) is doing some consulting work part-time. A friend since the late 1940s has gotten a patent on a manufacturing process and is working on a test device which requires much attention, many helpers, and many written reports. This can be a good experience or a bad experience depending on the results that day."

"What do you do for recreation? Do you have any hobbies?"

"Our recreation for body, mind, and spirit is inseparable from our work. We are on a flexible schedule here and whether we are playing or working may depend on who is defining the activity. One activity is mainly for pleasure, however, and that is feeding the birds and other hungry creatures. Every day in the late afternoon, I take out food, less in the summer and fall, more in the winter and spring.

"The crows get whole shelled corn and scratch feed, and near the house I fill half-coconut shells installed on the trees with raw peanuts, scratch feed, black sunflower seed, and wild birdseed. I put handfuls on the ground and on the balcony, and I smear peanut butter on certain trees. The number and variety of birds awaiting my afternoon performance is amazing to see. An indigo bunting bird was yesterday's surprise. If I am late, I get many vocal reminders becoming more and more demanding from irate customers. In addition to birds, we see many squirrels, frequent rabbit visitors, and some flying squirrels, deer, possums, terrapins, skunks, and foxes.

"We like taking short trips and go now and then to the nearby Smoky Mountains—especially to see deer, bears, turkeys, and other wildlife at Cades Cove, and to enjoy the breathtaking scenery from Look Rock. The views are magnificent and remind us that we have loved this place since childhood. On a clear day we can see the mountains from our home, but the close-up views are special."

"Are you active in a local church?"

"Yes. We are Presbyterians by heritage and upbringing and we joined Highland Presbyterian Church in Maryville. We felt welcomed there and we had family and friends in the congregation. Also we found the minister kind and caring. We have not taken on major responsibilities at the church, but we have done some short-term duties. We helped to refinish two pews, cleaned old bricks, and Bill designed the wrought-iron railing for the porch. He also checked the installation of the air-conditioning unit for the 'Old Mansion' portion of Highland Church. We have also contributed funds. During the work projects, we made new friends and accomplished needed improvements for the church."

"How is your health in retirement?"

"Well, at age seventy-five, we have physical problems that affect us at times. We have doctors who we think are capable, and we follow their advice. My mind and spirit seem to cooperate best when I feel good. There are days when forward progress is impossible. This is a good time to read, watch videos, do handwork, and relax. I thank God that my sons, and my husband, are no longer riding motorcycles in California traffic, as they once did."

"*I understand you still like to entertain guests from other countries in your home, just as you did when living in York. Is that true?*"

"Yes. We have had a series of guests who are/were students of Maryville College. Some are from the CELL program, which has classes for international students studying English as a second language. When Maryville College closes the dormitories for Christmas Holidays, Spring Break, or between sessions, the foreign students need a place to stay. We first called in to ask if there were 'country-loving students' who wished to stay with us, but now *they call us*!

"One guest was an interesting Japanese middle-school retired teacher who was (gasp!) fifty-five years old. His age did not alarm us. He was very happy to be served green tea, rice in a rice bowl with chopsticks—and he enjoyed the turkey too, since he was here Thanksgiving week. Christmas found us first with two Korean students; then one flew off to New York to visit relatives while another Korean student took her place. The next day (December 23), a young Malaysian family of five arrived. Haniza, the young mother, was one of our first international students in 1983 (I think).

"Haniza met her husband-to-be in Knoxville, Tennessee, when he was an engineering student at the University of Tennessee. We were overjoyed to see them and meet their bright, well-behaved children—ages eight, six, and twenty months. We had a wonderful Christmas together. The next day the visiting family left and one of the Korean girls went to visit others. Only one of the Korean girls was here for the 'big snowstorm' which delayed Maryville College classes for a day. This allowed her to arrive back at school on time even though our driveway had been blocked by snow.

"In February our last year's exchange student from Tokyo, Mika, arrived. Mika had completed her university courses and had worked two jobs to earn enough money to buy her own ticket to Maryville for her last long vacation before starting her permanent work. She has many friends at the college and was in and out for three weeks. We had much good Japanese food, most of which she had brought from Tokyo, and now prepared for us. Two days after Mika left for home, we had two new friends come for a week's visit. One student had been at the college a month, the other only a week. Their English was difficult, but we knew it was much better than our Korean."

"What do you consider the biggest challenge you have faced in retirement?"

"Our biggest challenge was caring for Bill's mother during the last years of her life. She was very ill when Bill brought her to York from her home in Knoxville, Tennessee. Her problem was congestive heart failure. She accepted the diet and medications prescribed for her but she hated getting older. After seven years, we had to take her to a nursing home. It was difficult for her and for us. She died six months later at age ninety-one."

"What advice would you give someone planning to retire?"

"I usually don't give advice unless someone asks me for it, but if they did, I would be happy to share our retirement experience and encourage them to enjoy life, and try to help God's creatures: birds, animals, and most of all, humans, as Bill and I have tried to do.

"1996 is a banner year for us. By year's end we will each have celebrated our seventy-fifth birthday as well as our fiftieth year of marriage. We have been richly blessed."

Helping Others
and Overcoming Great Loss

RHODA IYOYA

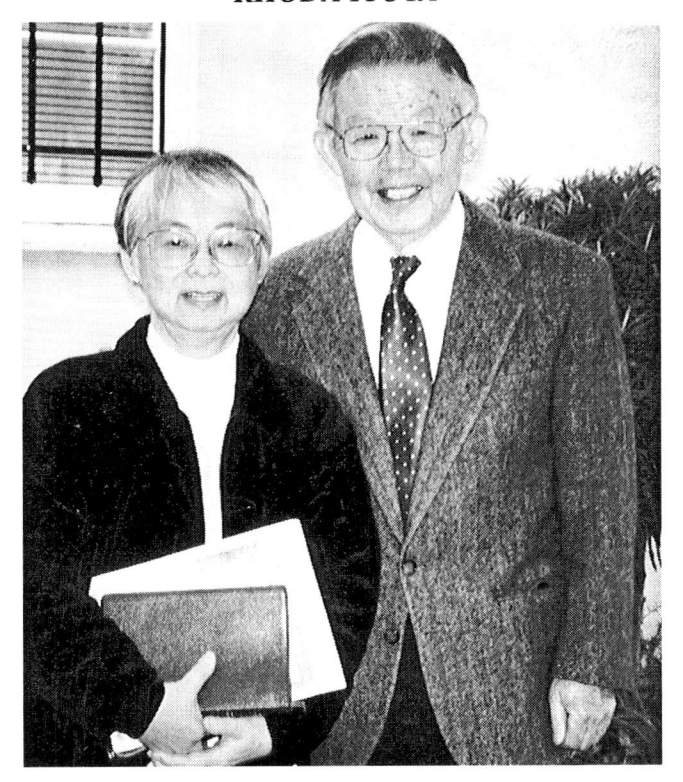

"How did retirement begin for you, Rhoda?"

"Well, my retirement years began in 1980 when I retired from public school teaching. I took early retirement at age fifty-five in order to take on a new challenge—to go to Japan as a fraternal worker for the Presbyterian Church, U.S.A., with my husband, Nick." Smiling gently, Rhoda continued.

"In Japan, we were assigned to be codirectors of the Serendipity Community Center in Iwakuni, Japan—a Christian Center sponsored by the National Council of Churches, U.S.A. and the National Council of Churches, Japan. The center served the U.S. Service personnel and their families in an off-base setting as well as the Japanese whose lives were affected by the presence of the American military. One of my main projects there was to start an enabling ministry for Japanese wives and fiancées of American service personnel.

"I had an English class for an intergenerational class in a local Japanese church. We struggled with <u>idioms</u>. One day I walked into class and was greeted by one of the senior members of the class with 'What's up?' There was an eight-year-old boy from another church who was terminally ill with leukemia. His one dream was to learn to speak English. His wonderful Christian spirit as he battled the disease was a source of inspiration. We played word games and had a wonderful time as he learned to speak English.

"*What other things were included in your program?*"

"Well, with the help of two bilingual Japanese staff members, we had an ongoing program of counseling and classes for Japanese wives and fiancées of American military personnel. In emergency situations we were there to help. For example, a woman whose husband had been returned to the U.S. and was desperately lonesome could not make the necessary arrangements to go overseas to join him. In her desperation, she took an overdose of sleeping pills and then came to the center for help. She needed immediate medical attention, followed by counseling. We helped to get the necessary paperwork done and intervened for her with base officials in English in order to make the arrangements to join her husband. As we sought help for others in similar circumstances, the base officers began to see the problems and both the chaplain's office and the family service office on base began to work cooperatively with us.

"*What kind of cultural problems did you have to deal with?*"

"One example is that Americans speak directly, whereas Japanese are 'circular,' speaking around a subject in an indirect way. Japanese wives not knowing English and also not knowing that there is a difference in how you express yourself in American culture compounded the problem of communication. The Japanese women struggled with these differences in our English classes.

"What about differences in food and eating habits?"

"Cooking was never my forte," said Rhoda, with a little laugh, "but I found myself giving basic American cooking lessons. Each Thanksgiving the wives helped in the preparation of an American Thanksgiving dinner with pumpkin pies, candied yams, vegetables, and salad, and invited the Japanese community to join us. Few Japanese have ever had a turkey dinner. We were able to purchase turkeys through the base, but the problem came when we tried to find an oven large enough to roast the turkeys—there were no Japanese ovens that large. One year, one of the soldiers who was a cook on base managed to roast our turkeys in the base ovens. Other years some American officers befriended us and roasted the turkeys in their home ovens—somehow, we managed. And the Japanese wives were introduced to an American holiday dinner and how to prepare it.

"Our three years in Japan were very meaningful ones, and we treasure the friendships we made during those years."

"Why did you return to the U.S.A. after three years in Japan?"

"We returned to the U.S. so Nick could assume one more pastorate before his retirement—followed by two interim pastorates. As a retiree, I was able to help him in his ministry and continue to pursue my interest in women's advocacy work and Christian Education work through the local church—as well as through the denomination."

"I understand you had a very close relationship with your parents. Could you share something about that relationship?"

"Yes. My parents have had a deep and abiding influence throughout my life, even in retirement. I have always had a tremendous respect for both of them. My father, Reverend Masamoto Nishimura, was a very gentle, committed, and unassuming man. He was very fair and very just. As a pastor, and because of his Christian commitment, he felt all people were equal in God's sight and as children of God deserved equal treatment, and he passed no judgment. He was chaplain to the Japanese prisoners in San Quenton and so often they were paroled in his care. They came and stayed with us and had their first meal with us. My father treated them in the same way he treated anyone else and expected us to do the same.

"My mother, Kimiko, was led to Christ through the Salvation Army in Japan. And because of that she was always a doer and responded readily to human need. That was another reason why our house was always filled with people. She was a woman ahead of her times and was an ardent advocate for women. She saw to it that I received the same educational privileges as my three brothers. She had the same expectations of me as of my brothers. At the same time she felt that we had to have fun in life. She took us fishing, camping, to new places, and she saw to it that we had swimming and music lessons. She told us it was important to have a variety of experiences so that we could enjoy life.

"In retirement, as I draw on what I learned from her, and savor and enjoy the retirement years, I'm very grateful to her for sharing with me her spirit of adventure. I sincerely believe that we prepare ourselves throughout our lifetime for the retirement years—when we have more leisure time.

"My parents were risk takers. In retirement they traveled the forty-eight states visiting their Japanese friends and raising funds to build retirement apartments for the Issei (first generation) adjacent to their church in Boyle Heights. Before my mother died, she saw their dream fulfilled. Later the Japanese community worked together to start the much more inclusive Japanese retirement homes in Boyle Heights.

"My parents were also people of prayer. The image of both of them sitting at the breakfast table with a cup of coffee and an open Bible each morning still is vivid in my memory. I too enjoy that morning coffee—and that morning devotional period has also become a meaningful part of our lives.

"*When did you come to the Monte Vista Grove retirement community in Pasadena, California?*"

"We first came here in September 1994," responded Rhoda, "after two years in an interim ministry in Ogden, Utah. With Nick at age seventy-two and I at sixty-eight, we finally fully retired. We sold our home in Seaside, California, and moved here. We were able to share in the building of a new duplex as 'builder-donors.' We enjoy our home, we enjoy the people who share life with us here, and we enjoy the security of knowing that we will be well cared for here for the rest of our lives. And our five grown children are happy to know that we are comfortable in our home and will be well cared for here.

"Two of our children live within half an hour of us and we are able to spend much time with them. The other three children and their spouses and our four grandchildren live in Northern California. We are able to see them at least six times a year. The time spent with all of them gives us much joy. Our children are now truly our best friends. Recently, our daughter who lives in our area said that she wanted her dad to share with her what he has learned through a lifetime of Bible study. Now we have an animated family Bible study two to three times a month, and Nick is so happy and pleased to be able to do this."

"How is your health now?"

"Both Nick and I are blessed with good health, with Nick now age seventy-four and I seventy. In order to maintain that health, we keep a regular schedule of exercise and diet. Each morning we spend half an hour each on the Nordic Track [exercise machine]; then I swim forty laps in our medium-size pool here while Nick does stretching exercises. This we do all year around when we are home. We walk and hike at other times. We eat simply, avoiding rich foods (except when we attend those scrumptious church potluck dinners).

"What do you do in your church and community?"

"Well, we enjoy life in our church. We help tutor at the local elementary school, assisting students who need a little extra help. I continue my interest and concern to share the 'Good News' with people of Japanese ancestry through the Japanese Presbyterian churches. I have been working on the Gospel Sharing Task Force and also on an internship project, which provides an internship experience in a Japanese-American Presbyterian church for a seminary student interested in ministry among the Japanese. Presently, I am on the board of the National Church Women United Executive Committee working for issues which affect the quality of life for women—especially for women who live on the fringes of society. This keeps me on my toes and active on my computer. It also means traveling across the country three to four times a year.

"Nick and I participate in the Elderhostel program and enjoy gaining new insights and making new friends. We try to make one big trip a year. Last year we went to Switzerland. This year we will be going to London and then to Turkey and Greece on a study trip titled 'Following in the Steps of St. Paul.' Our friends here tell us to do our traveling while our legs are strong and we are able."

"*What was the greatest challenge you have faced in retirement?*"

"Well, the death of our son really tested us. And it came so unexpectedly. While we were in Japan, our best letter-writer was our youngest son John ('Bodie') who was in his fourth year at Vassar College. He had visited us once in Japan. Because he knew how much we enjoyed getting mail in Japan, he often filled our mailbox with fun letters. In his last letter to us he described his new sport, rock climbing: 'There is a very intense feeling when you are on the rocks. It is very scary and yet also thrilling. When you are stuck two hundred feet off the ground it just gets more intense because there is almost no way to get down. Don't worry, though Mom. It is a very safe sport. It's almost safer than swimming.' With that assurance, I didn't worry. In fact, he had never given me cause to worry.

"And so when my brother called us early in the morning on November 8, 1982 to tell us that Bodie had taken his life, we couldn't believe it—not our Bodie. He loved life so much and lived it with such zest. He was a giving and compassionate person. He was a special friend of little children. He always brought that extra sparkle and sunshine into our lives. I felt like I had been struck down and completely drained of life. . . . at that moment when I received the news something inside me died—it was utter despair, hopelessness . . . I tried to pray . . . but how do you pray at a time like that? . . . . All I could say was 'God, please help us. . . give us the strength to go on living, especially for the sake of the remaining five children.'. . . We left Japan immediately. I can still remember that lonely plane ride, repeating the words of the twenty-third Psalm 'though I walk through the valley of the shadow of death, Thou art with me.'

"John loved Vassar College. It just seemed right to have his memorial service in the chapel, which had been important in his life there. Although we had planned a private service, the chaplain asked that we open it to the students. . . . they needed it as much as we did. . . . The students provided a spacious, beautiful home for our family and prepared meals for us. The memorial service planned by John's friends with the chaplain was a moving and meaning-filled celebration of John's life.

"Surrounded by so much warmth and support, sharing together that which was so good and beautiful in John's life for that moment gave us much strength and encouragement. We really felt God's presence in our lives—giving us a glimmer of hope. As we left the chapel, his classmates passed out daisies—their way of affirming life. I had experienced the overwhelming love of God expressed tangibly by his people. Although we found it difficult to verbalize our prayers, there was a community of believers praying for us. All this gave me sustenance for the difficult months ahead—I could physically begin to feel release from the weight of despair.

"This experience was shared by each member of our family—each in our own way. The months following were painful. It could have torn our family apart. And yet, through God's grace, I can say that miraculously we still enjoy the love and support of our family—and family means a great deal to us.

"When we live through such a crisis, we don't survive intact. We come through a different person. We have experienced a death of a part of ourselves in the death of Bodie, but we were not destroyed—we were in fact made strong—through Christ we were born anew.

"Those who prayed for me, who cared for me, forgave, and nurtured me in Christ's name helped me grow through suffering—finding a vital and living faith which gives me trust, meaning, and hope for the future. I have been able to become a more open channel for the healing love of God to flow through me into the hurting and brokenness which is all around me. I have been able to learn how to laugh at myself, and with others. I am learning to celebrate with aliveness and joy the gift of life—with all its mystery and wonder, absurdity, joy, and pain.

"Now I can accept that gift of being able to wake each morning, expectantly—able to live each day with gratitude, one day at a time. I don't look far into the future. I don't know what the years ahead hold, or how many years I still have. For, as the Bible says, 'Do not be anxious about tomorrow, for tomorrow will be anxious for itself. Let the day's own trouble be sufficient for the day.' (Matthew 6:34).

"The Bible also reminds me that 'Those who trust in the Lord for help will find their strength renewed. They will rise on wings like angels. They will run and not get weary. They will walk and not grow weak' (Isaiah 40:31).

"For all this I give God thanks and praise."

Does a Housewife Retire?

DOT HORCHER

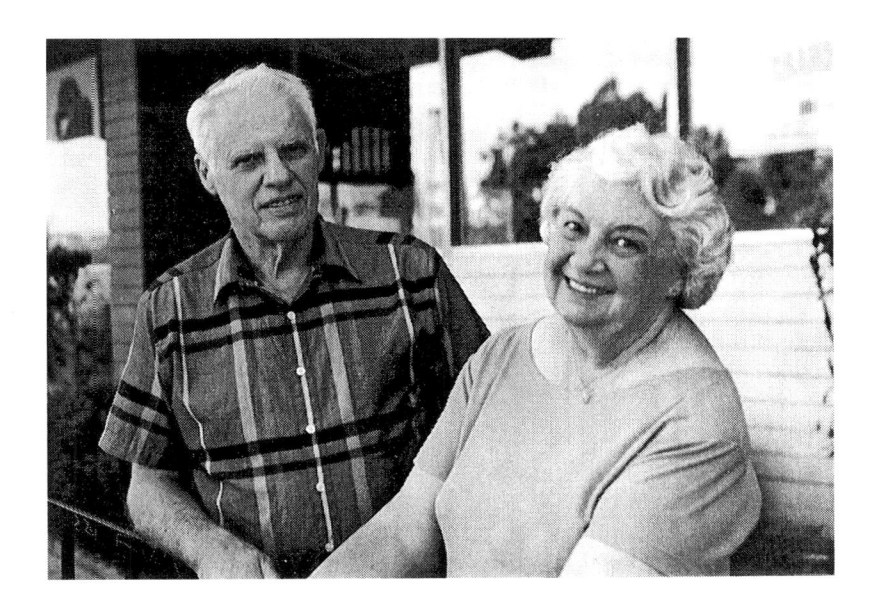

"*What do you mean when you say your retirement is different from others?*"

"Well, did I retire? I don't think so, certainly not in the professional sense for I was and am the 'once and future housewife' (retired or not). My husband, George, actually retired, and when he did, both our lives changed.

"Last week, George and I visited our son, Charles, and his young family in their small home in the Tehachapi Mountains. This late in May there weren't many wildflowers still blooming except Farewell-to-Spring. That is a wistful, sweet/sad name for a simple weedy plant with pale orchid blossoms.

"This, and another wildflower I will mention later, set me to thinking about the seasons of my life. Although I said farewell to my personal springtime long ago, those early years are evergreen in memory and for the most part, they are sweet to recall.

"I must have been 'born lucky' for I was cherished by a full set of parents and grandparents, all of them churchgoers. During the summer of my tenth year, I was baptized in a river (although there was a baptistery in our church) because I wanted to do everything 'just like Jesus.'

"After being immersed and raised up from the water, I saw the beauty of the sky looking iridescent in late afternoon and a crowd of people standing in front of dark pine trees, singing 'Yes! We'll gather at the river, the beautiful, the beautiful river, gather with the saints at the river, that flows by the throne of God.' That springtime of my life memory remains keenly focused and precious to me." A joyous smile brightened Dot's face as she recalled this happy event.

"Tell me about your family."

"I met my husband after a year in college. Through a scholarship I attended a Presbyterian school, Trinity University, in Waxahachie, Texas (now in San Antonio) for a year. Later, when I met this blue-eyed boy on July 4, 1942, and he told me he was a lifelong Presbyterian—well, that seemed an added attraction—not that he needed one! George and I were married the following summer, July 3, 1943, in Cambridge, Massachusetts, where he was being trained as a naval radar officer.

"We were living in Lawrence, Kansas when I formally joined the Presbyterian Church and our two children, Ruth and Charles, were baptized. It was then that a friend introduced me to Presbyterian Women, through a social group called 'Presbytery-Anns.'

"I won't push the metaphorical seasons of my life here except to say that the time came when I was deep into 'summer'—and I never even knew when it began. We had another son, Paul, baptized as an infant."

"My wife tells me you do a lot of church work. Tell me about that."

"Well, my busy years of work and responsibility, coupled with a thin wallet and related woes, sent me stumbling into the Women of the Church in the 1950s. I wasn't worth much to the organization, being inexperienced, undereducated, and with no overwhelming natural talents. Nevertheless, I found a warm welcome and good friends. It was the beginning of a long, rewarding adventure for me and I am thankful for it. All these decades later I am still able to serve the church through the Presbyterian Women.

"I am now completing three years as vice moderator of Presbyterian Women of the Presbytery of San Gabriel near my home in Diamond Bar, California. Yes, I am their program chairperson and believe it or not, I asked for this difficult job because it is the work I like best. (George kids me, 'Shake your head—I wanna hear the marbles rattle!') In addition to women's work (local, presbytery, and synod levels at different times), I have taught Sunday school, served as an 'elder' and on one 'pastor-seeking' committee.

"Until George retired, almost all the above jobs were interrupted when he would get a foreign job assignment (he worked for a multinational engineering corporation), and I would joyfully tag along—to England and to South Africa. After George's retirement, we were needed many times to help our extended family. Part of that was helping our three remaining parents through their final sad and lonely years. We also lend a hand occasionally with our grandkids: eight of them, now aged twenty-five to three. I learned to tailor my work for the church so that it could proceed without my physical presence, when necessary.

"I guess 'summer' had become 'autumn,' for sometimes I felt awfully blue, useless, and far removed from the idealistic child who had promised to 'be like Jesus,' and gloried in her baptism. I wondered if God had lost track of me and I prayed that I might be given worthwhile work to do. My church invited people to participate in a 'prayer chain' and I volunteered to be a link. I haven't been A-plus faithful—sometimes I was a *missing* link. Even so, this is privileged work and I treasure it."

"How is your health?"

"It was good until 1988. It seems that most of us request prayer when health is threatened. During the summer of 1988 (one of my pivotal years), my own good health was knocked off center by a severe case of shingles. The attack came while George and I were visiting my parents at their ranch home on the west bank of the Nueces River, forty miles north of Uvalde, Texas. It was a trying time—perhaps I triggered my illness by trying too hard to be all that my parents and sister, my husband, and my children (and especially myself) wanted—and needed—me to be.

"The ranch was beautiful that year. Ample rains had cleaned and filled the river and turned the rangeland green. Ancient oak and giant pecan trees gave cooling shade to the house and provided food, shelter, and romping room for birds and squirrels. We took our morning coffee to the screened 'river porch' and waited quietly to see deer go down to the river to drink. It was a lovely time and sweet to remember. But suddenly, I was in great pain—pain such as I had never known before, around-the-clock and brutal.

"I was determined not to exceed the doctor's prescribed dosage of strong pain medicine: one pill every four hours. I continued to cook for George and my father and help take care of my pitifully diminished little mother during the daytime, but during the nights pain would awaken me with a mule-kick jolt—and there would be two hours to wait until pill time.

"Hoping not to disturb those who slept, I would go quietly to the river porch, build myself a nest of pillows in an old sling-back canvas beach chair, snap a symphony into my little cassette player, plug in the earphones, and let music do its soothing work. When the tape was played and I sat alone in the darkness of the small hours, I became aware of a companion, one also sleepless—an owl which had returned from her night's journey to tuck in and rest in her treehouse.

"I never made a sound but she knew I was there, listening, and she always gave me a soft, sleepy hoot-hoot salute before she slept. Was this a form of prayer?—a comforting gift from the Holy Spirit, who never sleeps, yet knows that we must and cares that we do? I only know that I cherish the memory.

"After we returned to our home in California, our daughter came to live with us for a while, until she could get on her feet financially. Ruthie was a great help to me, taking over the heavy cleaning and supporting me in meal preparation. We enjoyed a good green salad every suppertime (thanks to Ruthie) and learned to eat half-raw (well, maybe I should say half-cooked) vegetables. And I began a satisfying, grandmother-type hobby. I began to collect and read the Newberry Award—winning books written for children since 1922—all good stories, and not a cussword in a carload! On July 3, 1993, George and I celebrated our fifty years of 'wedded bliss' with a dinner for family and friends. Another celebration was an automobile trip around the U.S.A.—visiting the many places where we had lived."

"What has been your greatest challenge (other than shingles) since reaching retirement age?"

"That would be my tangle with politics. In November 1994, our son Paul was elected to his third term to the California Assembly in Sacramento. Although he thought of himself as a Republican in the Lincoln tradition, Paul had become disillusioned with what he saw, heard, and experienced among Republicans then in power. The load on his conscience was proving indigestible, so Paul re-registered as 'Decline to State' (independent), and when it was time to cast his vote for Speaker of the Assembly, Paul voted, not for the designated Republican, but for the person he believed to be all-around better for the job, Mr. Willie Brown, a Democrat. Then, an explosion of troubles began for us.

"Many of our friends and family didn't know what on earth to say, so they became very quiet. Others closed ranks around us, to comfort and uphold. Strangers called, some out of curiosity, others to question and denounce. Some were people who sought us out to praise our son's courage and to help Paul resist the recall election that was scheduled for May, 1995. It was hard to see our good German name Horcher ("to listen" was George's dad's translation) corrupted into W-H-O-R-E-C-H-E-R—lettered onto crude placards and paraded on television.

"It was difficult to see our dear son made the object of cheap, mean jokes. It was even harder to learn that some old friends joined the campaign to recall Paul (no one in the California Legislature had been recalled in over eight decades).

"One night the phone rang and a man's voice said, 'Mrs. Horcher, we want to post security guards at your home.' I supposed he had mistaken me for Paul's wife, but he insisted I was the one he had called to warn. He said anonymous calls had come in saying, 'We can't get to you, Paul Horcher—you are too well-guarded—but we know where your parents live.' Click!

"We are easy to find. We are in the phone book; we live on an open, two-way street. Soon, a succession of strong, quiet, armed men began parking their cars curbside at our house, around-the-clock, for several weeks. December nights were cold and I worried about those men, keeping a lonely vigil to protect us and let us sleep safely. Early in the morning I took hot coffee to them, before I had my first cup. And I offered them hot bricks at night, to help keep warm. They just smiled at me and told me they were used to it and came prepared.

"Those good men never let us out of their sight—they even went to church with us. They stopped everyone who came to our door, and they intercepted the postman to check our mail. One day a small box arrived. It was wrapped in plain brown paper and had an interesting rattle. The on-duty guard who rang our doorbell held the package at arm's length and implored, 'Please tell me you know someone in Florida named Maggie Penny.' It was a box of harmless seashells I had requested. Ironically, the small seashells were for decorating name tags for a women's program I had titled 'A Safe House.'

"Despite heroic efforts made by Paul and many other good people whom I shall love forever, Paul was recalled. We had never been prouder of our children than we were for the way they handled defeat. Paul took it like a hero, never whining once, and his wife, his brother, and his sister all stood by him. I call that *character*—and I rejoice to see it in our children.

"Finally, I realized it would be necessary for me to declare a general amnesty within my troubled spirit—and so I have. Now I can get on with my life, with forgiveness for all and with true affection for many. That's a blessing and I believe my life's scale is heavily weighted toward the *blessings* side. I hope that what I have written here will let some of that holy light shine through the common everyday words I have used."

"*How do you view the future?*"

"Well, having gone past the Biblical 'three-score and ten' years, I suppose I have entered the 'winter' of my life. The word winter always brings to mind C.S. Lewis' wonderful idea from his *Narnia Chronicles*, how the magnificent lion Aslan (Christ) had come ashore in Narnia (the kingdom of—your choice) to break the evil spell there, where it was 'always winter, but never Christmas.'

"Recently a stranger told me that in Russia, elderly, white-headed women are called 'God's dandelions.' When I repeated that to my young granddaughters, they immediately began to blow on my gray hair, trying to blow me bald-headed." (See J. Barrie Shepherd's poem, "Hope Weed," for a view of the dandelion as a resurrection symbol—always coming back.)

"When I was with George in South Africa, I had to adjust to Christmas coming in their summer and Easter in autumn, not in springtime. I had to recognize that Jesus Christ is not confined to a season, a country, a political party, a race, a class, or an age, but for *all*. Hallelujah!

Surviving and Serving in Retirement

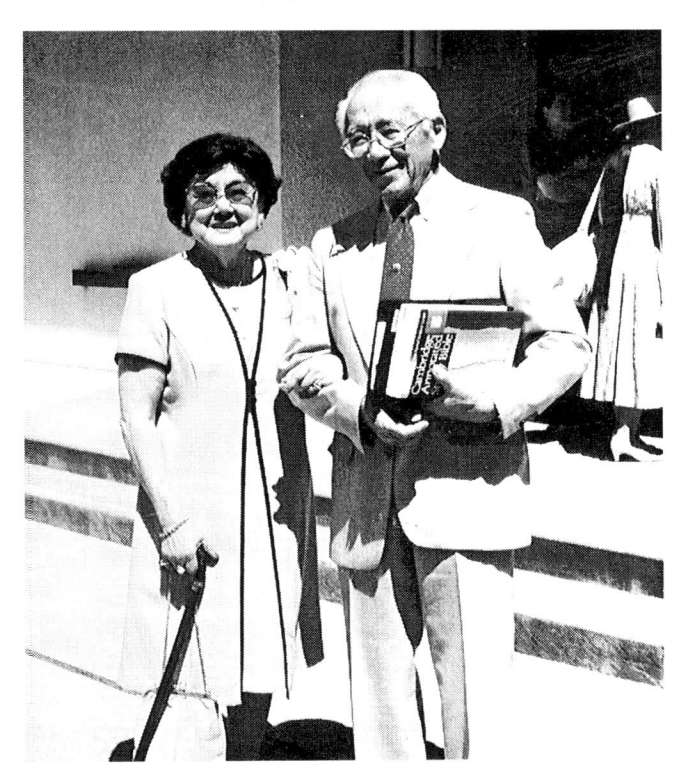

TED TAJIMA

"*Ted, I understand your retirement began in a rather unusual way.*"

"Yes. It was not a dark and stormy night, but it was a strange one that led to my retirement back in March, 1983. My wife, Setsu, and I had settled down to a quiet evening, she with a magazine and I with papers to correct—the usual task for a high school teacher.

"About nine o'clock we got a frantic call from our daughter Elaine, whose three-year-old Aimee had fallen, banged her head against a patio door, and could not stop bleeding. We rushed Aimee to the emergency hospital, admitted her, then waited an interminable time for her cut to be attended to. The emergency room was crowded, unusually I thought for a weeknight. After waiting almost two hours, I stood up and headed for a coffee machine.

"I didn't take a step before fainting and falling prone to the floor. Then ironically it wasn't Aimee who was rushed in to an examining room in an emergency. I was. Examinations disclosed that I was bleeding internally from stomach cancer, and in five days, an early cancer growth was removed from my stomach." With a wry smile and in an amazingly energetic voice, Ted continued.

"Someone must have been watching over me. Sharing in Aimee's emergency led to the discovery of my cancer in time to remove it. Three months later, after thirty-five years of public school teaching, I decided that cancer surgery was telling me something, and I retired at age sixty-one."

"How has retirement worked out for you?"

"Retirement has been far from boring. There was much to look forward to, and there was so much that my wife and I did not expect. For example, learning to live with each other twenty-four hours a day was a challenge, and a delight, in itself. While I was teaching, there were long days at school, where advising student journalists putting out a weekly newspaper led to late days every week. Then there were long hours correcting papers at night that led to neglecting my wife too many hours a night. So retirement meant doing things together, something I admit I'm still learning to do."

"Have you had any especially happy experiencees in retirement?"

"Oh, yes. One of the hopes and wishes of a retiree is to travel. This wish for us came true in a surprising way. At my retirement, former students got together and raised funds for a trip to Japan for Setsu and me. In October of that year we flew to Japan, our first trip abroad. We spent a wonderful five weeks enjoying the bustling cities, majestic mountains, and scenic ocean shorelines of Japan plus learning about the rich culture of our forefathers (and mothers). Best of all, we enjoyed meeting people all the way from cold Sendai in the north to pleasantly warm Nagasaki in the South. As you know, Nagasaki was famous for two events: It was the gateway for Christianity's first entry into Japan and the tragic site of the second atomic bomb.

"We also had five rainy days in exciting Hong Kong and visited the border of Red China. On our way home, we stopped for a leisurely, blissful week in Honolulu with my brother Tsuneo and his wife Bernice. It was an unforgettable trip, and we owe it to some great former students and friends who were really generous."

"What has been your greatest challenge in retirement?"

"That would be our family health problems. Setsu and I have been a real challenge to the medical profession and the medical insurance industry. She has suffered cardiac arrest and five major surgeries: mastectomy, arterial carotid vein operations, small intestines twice, and gallstones—in addition to glaucoma and cataract eye surgeries. In addition to the cancer problem, I have had kidney surgery. All in all, we have been taking care of each other in times of sickness and health—till that time we promised in our marriage vows.

"But these experiences have been more than a series of chores caring for each other. We have learned the need for love and attention, something I feel I have been remiss in exhibiting for the forty years of marriage before retirement.

"It has not been just the skill of wonderful surgeons we have come to know. We have had the love and care and prayers of family and friends, who have personalized the unending love that God has for us. We praise God that his people are our friends and caregivers."

"I know you have done a lot for your church in retirement. Please share some of that activity."

"In our church, I have found an opportunity to serve with what small talents I may have. Setsu and I owe much to the Church: some fifty-plus years ago we met while singing in the choir as teenagers. As they say, 'the rest is history.' In 1993 we celebrated our golden wedding anniversary, which is a story in itself. In brief, we had married in a small town in Ohio, to which we moved during World War II—and forced evacuation from California. There were only nine people at our wedding, which my father, the Reverend Kengo Tajima, performed.

"In 1993, Setsu felt—and I concurred—old friends were seeing each other usually at funerals. Also, we had never had a church wedding. Decision: we shall repeat our wedding vows in the presence of our daughters and grandchildren and relatives and friends. And we did, at First Presbyterian Church, Altadena, California, with three hundred guests we were unable to have in Chagrin Falls, that small town in Ohio where we married. Friends came from Chicago, Hawaii, Japan, and the great Northwest. It was a wonderful reunion for family and friends, the service was emotional, the dinner was delicious, the dancing was fun, and friends got to meet each other and enjoy. . .

"In our church I continued in retirement a service I had begun back in 1950, editing the weekly newsletter. This has continued to be a Monday night activity in retirement, perhaps to the consternation of readers who have borne with me these forty-six years since I first began. I have enjoyed the chance to serve our church and to communicate its ministry. Setsu, too, has shown tremendous patience for, lo, these many years, worrying about the late hours and whether or not I would finish each edition in time—let alone sharing the embarrassment when I made errors. She is also waiting for my second retirement, from editing the church papers.

"For the church there have been other opportunities to serve. In the Presbytery of San Gabriel, I served six years as a member of the nominations committee, a position that involved one meeting a month and gave me the opportunity to suggest others for Presbytery responsibilities. I have also served six years and am continuing to serve as secretary of the Board of Directors of the Ecumenical Council of Pasadena Area Churches.

"In this capacity I have had the opportunity of meeting and working with a number of active clergypersons and lay leaders from a variety of churches. This has been an enriching experience for me, giving me more insight into the community. As a commissioner to the General Assembly in 1994, I met clergy and lay leaders from all over the nation and the world, meeting to consider matters of the National Church and worshiping together.

"My most challenging work in my church is serving my third term as a 'ruling elder' on our Church Session (ruling body), which is responsible for planning and overseeing all church activities. My most pleasant church activity is singing in the church choir—yes, something begun in the late 1930s and still continuing in the 1990s. My only regret is that Setsu, whom I met in the choir as a teenager, is no longer able to sing with us. She has a beautiful soprano voice and we could certainly use her."

"*Don't you also teach English as a Second Language in retirement?*"

"Yes. I have had the opportunity to continue what I had done professionally in the U.S. Army and the public schools—teaching. For eight years, I have taught an intensive workshop in English for university students and teachers from the Kansai region of Japan. The class has given me the opportunity to do what I love, teach, and to meet young people from Nishinomiya, Kobe, and Osaka.

"The students come to Spokane, Washington, sister city to Nishinomiya, and the class meets for five weeks in a classroom of Spokane Falls Community College, where our oldest daughter is a dean. Field trips to business and commercial districts and to scenic sights, including a wheat farm—a rarity in Japan—make up activities outside the classroom. Working with young people has an invigorating effect. They make this teacher feel younger, certainly a serendipity of this work.

"Almost everyone who retires is asked the question, 'Well, how do you like retirement; what do you do to keep busy?' The answer? It would take too much time to answer fully, but I will say one thing. God, family, friends, and activities are enough to keep us out of mischief."

Overcoming Internment and a Handicap, to Serve

ARTHUR TSUNEISHI

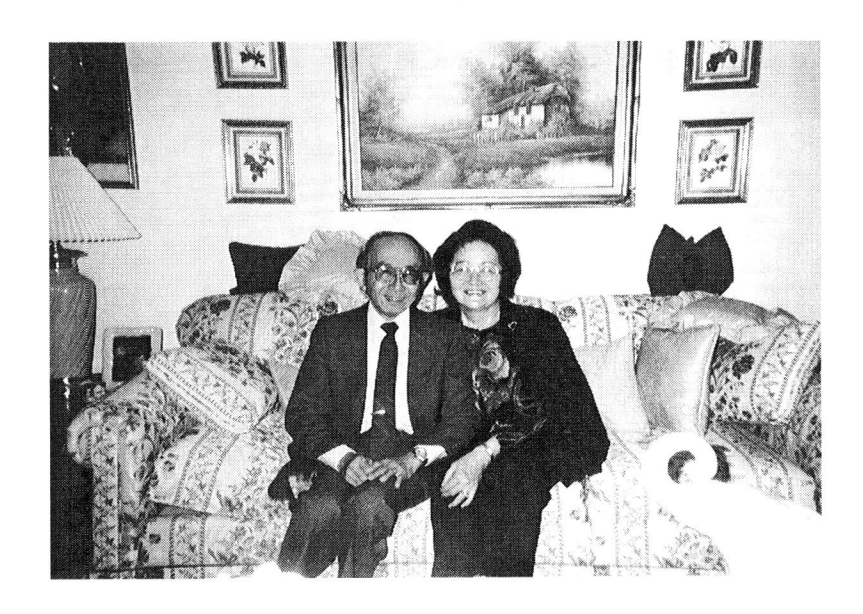

"I understand you were one of the Japanese-Americans put into an <u>internment camp</u> during World War II."

"Yes. I was attending Pasadena Junior College just prior to Pearl Harbor. When I first saw the Executive Order 9066 posted on Myrtle Avenue in Monrovia, California, I can still remember exclaiming, 'Hey, they can't do that to me, I'm an American citizen!' After that bitter experience, receiving the reparations legislated for us was a welcome validation of what this country is all about—honoring its citizens by trying to remedy its mistakes."

"*Wasn't it soon after that internment camp experience that you became partly paralyzed and had difficulty walking?*"

"Yes. I underwent a spinal operation in 1944 in Chicago, where I had relocated from the Heart Mountain internment camp in Wyoming—where our family was incarcerated. It left me seventy-five percent paralyzed in my lower extremities and thus the War Relocation Authority (WRA) sent me back to camp—but in Poston, Arizona, to recuperate since Heart Mountain, as well as Chicago, was too cold.

"It was there that I made a commitment to Christ, so I always give as my testimony the verses from Psalm 119:67 and 71—'that before I was afflicted, I went astray, but now I have kept thy word... It is good for me that I was afflicted that I might learn thy statutes.' Also I often share that 'if there is one positive thing that has come out of that incarceration, it was that I became a Christian in an American concentration camp!'"

"*I understand that in spite of your handicap you have not only served many years as a pastor but also continued some Christian work in your retirement.*"

"Yes. After pastoring churches in Honolulu, Los Angeles, San Diego, and San Lorenzo for thirty-six years, I spent the last four years before retirement as the English-speaking executive secretary of our Holiness Church Conference. (Our Conference began in 1920 in Los Angeles with a group of young Japan-born Bible students. We have churches in California as well as Hawaii today.) I retired fully in July 1993 at the age of seventy-two. My wife, Sally, and I retired in a home which I had purchased in 1974, along with one of my daughters who needed a place to teach piano.

"Since our retirement we have done 'pulpit supply' work, led Sunday school classes at times, [and] counseled people, and [we] still attend monthly pastors meetings—as well as our annual <u>General Conference</u>. Also we have served in an advisory capacity to our churches in Orange County, California, and in the San Gabriel, California, area.

"My wife, Sally, tutors our Chinese neighbor's children of elementary school age. They originally came from Vietnam, so I often assist in tutoring them as well. They are bright children, and they call us 'Grandma' and 'Grandpa.' Sally always gives them treats after their lessons. They like that. Five of our seven grandchildren live in Colorado Springs and one in the San Francisco Bay area. We visit them when we can."

"Didn't you also help a Vietnamese family get settled in America?"

"Yes. In 1975 when the Vietnamese refugees were just arriving at nearby Oakland Airport, we asked our congregation, 'How should we respond to sponsoring such a family?' That very week as a young Asian man walked by our church, I found out he had just come from Vietnam. He, along with three other adults and five children were all packed in one room of a motel nearby. We immediately took all of them into our home. Three of our eight children were still at home, so it made for a large 'extended' family for the next few months until we were able to find a home for them. Two of the men stayed with us longer.

"Through the years, we have conducted marriage ceremonies for several of the children, as well as some of the adults. We keep in contact with them, as they still consult us on various matters—since we are 'Mom' and 'Daddy' to them. When we visit our daughter and family in the Bay area, it is also to touch base with our Vietnamese family. It is heartening to see how well they have done: children graduating college, adults working mostly in the electronic field, and young marrieds buying homes."

"What traveling have you managed to do?"

"Well. Upon our 'retirement' from the pastorate in 1989, Sally and I took our second trip to Japan. Our first trip was in 1976. Alex Haley's *Roots* had just swept the country. To go to Japan and find our 'roots' was a most affirming experience. We knew we weren't 'Japanese' when we disembarked at the Tokyo Airport and lined up to be processed. We were told to line up in the 'foreigners' line. It was a joy to meet relatives for the first time and to reconnect with young farm trainees we had helped when they came to the U.S.A. in the 1950s and early 1960s. We had led many of them to Christ. One had studied at Tokyo Christian College and had become a pastor in Nagoya. On our second trip to Japan, he had moved out of the pastorate, but he and his wife were on the staff of a wonderful Christian senior citizen's facility called the King's Garden. We visited there and shared our testimony.

"One highlight on both trips to Japan was to visit Sally's relatives in the Amakusa area in Kumamoto. A graveside plot bordering the relative's farm revealed a unique gravestone on which we were told was a Christian marker. It turned out that it was a relative we believe had been martyred when Christianity came to Japan over four hundred years ago from Portugal. A nearby museum featured this relative who apparently was a part of the 'hidden Christian' movement, because of the severe persecution of Christians by the Japanese government.

"At Amakusa the Japanese children proudly shared at school about our visit. Also when we departed, one relative asked whether we would drop off some gifts to relatives in Hawaii, not comprehending that California and Hawaii are an ocean apart. Later, we visited national Christian workers we had supported for years."

"What exercise and recreation do you have in retirement?"

"Well, since I am limited in things like walking, which my wife does every morning, I work out daily on my exercise machine, which has been beneficial. In my retirement years, vegetable gardening has become an enjoyable pastime. I have the joy of seeing seeds I plant sprout, in various stages of growth, and then bear fruit. An added benefit is the good taste of vegetables we grow, which is much better than store-bought produce."

"What do you see as some of the blessings you have received in retirement?"

"Well, it may seem a small blessing but since our children have 'flown the coop' we have found 'Sainan,' a labrador dog, which we 'inherited' from one of our daughters who moved to Hawaii, a wonderful companion. My wife and I often comment, 'Sainan is almost human'—that is, with her responses and the ways she communicates her needs to us.

"Another godsend has been my Macintosh computer, which I purchased after my retirement from the pastorate. It was useful in writing memos, letters, and messages during the four years I served as an executive secretary. But I also found it such an enjoyable tool that I have been using it to write my memoirs for the benefit of my children and grandchildren. I'm still a neophyte in its use, so when I hear about the internet, it just boggles my mind!"

"What would you say is the basic theme of your many years of ministry?"

"Well, once my wife asked me 'What has been the bottom line of your years of ministry?' Off the top of my head, I responded with ideas like the number of churches we have pastored, the number of people we have led to Christ, using statistics. But, realizing that wasn't what she was fishing for, I asked her what she felt it was. She responded *'relationships!'* Finally it really hit me. Isn't that why we find in the Bible how God created us in his image and likeness? Why? Very obviously for fellowship. For relationship.

"In the Bible don't we find example after example about the importance of relationships? One example is Jesus' parable of the loving father who welcomed back the prodigal son. And didn't our Lord boil down all the commandments to just two? Namely, to love God with all our heart, soul, and mind, and to love our neighbor as ourself? With today's relationships so fractured in our families, in our churches, and in our politics, isn't the gospel of God's love for us and everyone the great antidote to our deep dilemma? Isn't love for God and others the key to becoming able to connect relationally in meaningful and loving ways?

"Recently, I have had to 'graduate' from the use of a cane and crutches to the occasional use of a wheelchair—yet at age seventy-five, I do feel strongly that God has blessed my ministry and continues to bless me and my family today."

Helping to Evangelize People, Near and Far

CHRISTY WILSON, JR

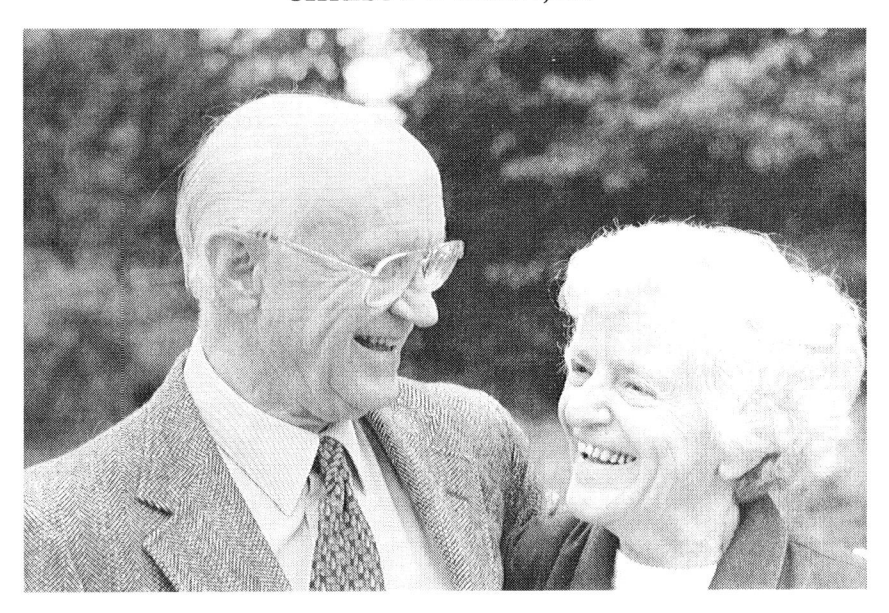

"*Your friend, Paul Hensley, refers to you and Betty as 'Mr. and Mrs. Tentmaker.' What does that mean?*"

"Well, Paul knows that my wife Betty and I served in a 'tentmaking' ministry in Afghanistan from 1951 to 1973, teaching English in a government school and trying to make a Christian witness at the same time. He also knows that in 1979 I published a book titled *Today's Tentmakers* based on Saint Paul's support of his ministry by making tents. That's why Paul Hensley gave us that gracious compliment." Christy seemed happy, but also a little embarrassed, at being complimented for his unusual work.

"Having played tennis with you, I am amazed at how healthy you seem to be at age seventy-four. How do you keep so healthy?"

"Saint Paul says our 'body is a temple of the Holy Spirit' and we should take care of our body. I try to take care of my body by eating healthful foods and exercising, but I know that my main source of strength is the Lord. Billy Graham has said that the weaker and older he gets, the more he needs to trust Christ's strength. Betty and I have found this to be true, too. This fits in with our Lord's words to the Apostle in II Corinthians 12:8, 'My grace is sufficient for you, for My power is made perfect in weakness.' I know I am growing older and weaker, but with the Lord's help, I manage to keep going."

"I admire the way you continue helping to evangelize people in retirement."

"It is biblical to do so. In Psalm 92:14 the psalmist said that believers 'will still bear fruit in old age,' and I'm trying to do that. In the Bible, the only ones who retired were the Levites at age fifty. The reason for this was that in their job of sacrificing animals, they had to lift heavy oxen and do other difficult tasks. But there were even exceptions for this. For example, Zechariah who became John the Baptist's father was 'well along in years.' But as a Levite he was chosen by lot to offer incense in the Temple.

"The Levites Moses and Aaron started their ministries at eighty and eighty-three, respectively. Thus, Betty and I have chosen to 'retire to active service' as long as we can. We believe that with Paul, we should continue to fight the good fight and finish the race, keeping the faith. Our God-given task is to help evangelize the world. And there are many more peoples . . . to be reached for Christ."

"I understand you have had a book published since retirement. Tell how that came about."

"One of my Chinese students was involved in that. I was given a great surprise on the occasion of my seventieth birthday—which was the age for retirement from Gordon-Conwell Theological Seminary in South Hamilton, Massachusetts, where I had taught for eighteen years. In China a person's seventieth birthday is considered the pinnacle of his or her life. One of my students from a Chinese background got tapes of my lectures in which I had told a lot of true stories. He and his wife put them into a word processor and on my birthday, without me knowing anything about it, they presented me with a laser printed desktop published book of one hundred forty-two pages of my stories.

"That book has been published and is called *More To Be Desired Than Gold*. It has sold over eleven thousand copies and has gone into three editions and is distributed by the Book Centre at Gordon-Conwell, 130 Essex Street, South Hamilton, Massachusetts 01982. All of the profits have gone for scholarships to help international students."

"*In addition to supporting you in your ministry, I know that Betty has been active in some things of her own. What have been some of her activities?*"

"Betty's activities are many. She has taught conversational English to refugees who have come to Southern California. She also teaches missions to the Sunday school children in our church. Besides this, she prays for and writes to Gordon-Conwell grads who are serving the Lord all around the world."

"*Do you keep in contact with people in tentmaking ministries today?*"

"Oh yes. Since retiring, I have been to conferences on tentmaking in Brazil, in Chiang Mai in Thailand, in Seoul, Korea, and in different parts of the United States. I still try to encourage Christians with the idea of tentmaking. As Dr. Elton Trueblood said, 'We need a second Reformation. In the first one, the people of God were given the word of God. Now we need one where the people of God are given the work of God.'"

"*What do you see as the future hope for a mission to Muslims?*"

"That is a challenging goal. Since I was born in a Muslim country, in Tabriz, Iran, where my parents were missionaries, and since Betty and I spent twenty-two years in Afghanistan, we are very concerned to seek to reach Muslims for Christ. With the Zwemer Institute of Muslim Studies in Pasadena needing a director, I was invited after retirement to serve in this position for six months. Just as we are seeing the collapse of Communism in much of the world, so I believe through prayer we will see the walls around Muslim nations and hearts come down. The Bible states, 'The weapons of our warfare are not carnal but are mighty through God to pulling down of strongholds, casting down vain imaginations and every high thing that exalts itself against the knowledge of God' (II Cor. 10:4,5).

"Betty and I have also enjoyed attending the Sunday evening services at the Anaheim Vineyard. John Wimber has given us a prophecy that we will reach Muslims through 'signs and wonders,' some of which are seen at his services there. This has been a great encouragement for us to keep praying and working among followers of the Islamic faith—not only in the States but also abroad.

"Thus I have traveled to Central Asia and have worked with Christians who are serving there. Since people in that part of the world have so much eye trouble, while serving in Kabul, Afghanistan, we built an eye hospital and an institute for the blind. This pattern is now being reproduced in other nations of Central Asia. Also, Betty and I were invited to go to Pakistan to attend a conference of those who were working with Afghan people—especially Afghan refugees."

"I understand you have been named 'honorary director' of the fiftieth anniversary celebration of the InterVarsity Missionaries Convention at Urbana, Illinois in December 1996."

"Yes. Betty and I have been invited to participate in that 'Golden' anniversary. It was at the first one held at the University of Toronto in 1946 that Betty and I first met. Dr. Ralph Winter who has started the U.S. Center for World Mission was also a student there. He has produced a course which is called 'Perspectives on the World Christian Movement.' This helps follow up with students who make the commitment to serve as missionaries. I have had the opportunity to teach sessions of this course in many churches and schools across the country.

"The greatest investment that we have is our lives. It is a privilege to invest them for Christ and the glory of God for as long as we can. As the Bible says, 'Whatever you do, do all for the glory of God.' This is the reason Betty and I have retired to active service—especially the effort to evangelize people near and far."

Retirement: An Enjoyable Phase of Life

BOB AND PEGGY THURMAN

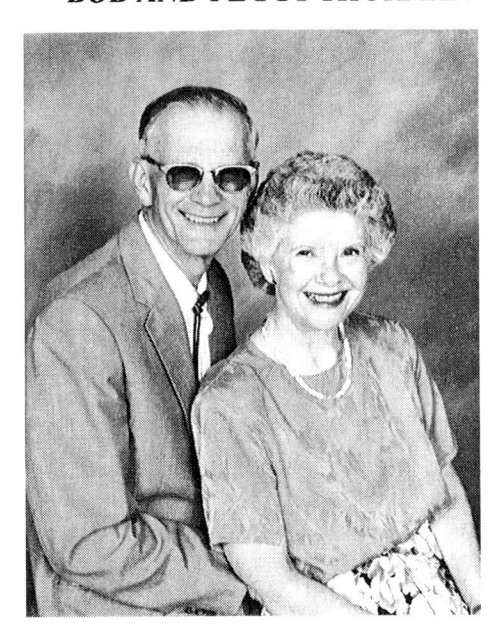

"How did you plan for retirement?"

"For me, retirement is another phase of my life—just as going into the army, being married, changing professional directions, and becoming a grandfather were phases. I looked forward to it just as I looked forward to the other phases—no regrets, no fears, great anticipation.

"I was a professor in early childhood education at the University of Tennessee for twenty-seven years. Colleagues often approached retirement with less than great enthusiasm since, they said, they did not know what they would do because teaching was their major interest. With that in mind, I began planning for retirement years before the event. But what would I do after retirement?

"Dr. Paul Tournier, the Christian Swiss psychiatrist, provided part of the answer. He wrote that people who continued the same kind of work as a volunteer that they had done for pay had not retired, only changed jobs. To retire meant moving into different activities. For me that meant enjoying reading, listening to music, hiking, photography, storytelling, searching family history and photos, writing, and working in the yard—especially being active in my church and enjoying time with our family." Tall, slim Bob smiled as he presented the activities he enjoyed in retirement.

"At what age did you decide to retire?"

"I debated that question. Should I take early retirement at age sixty-two or wait until sixty-five? The answer came when I served as visiting professor at a college in Oregon in 1984 to 1985. My professional responsibilities were few and I had time to pursue personal interests. My wife, Peggy, and I found we could live on much less money and still have a full, interesting life. I knew I was ready to retire.

"When I learned the University did not have a plan for early retirement, I developed one. The department head took it to appropriate administrators who approved it and I decided to retire in December 1990 at age sixty-two.

"We then bought five acres in Blount County that had woods, wildlife, and a beautiful view of the Smoky Mountains. We built a home and moved there in the fall of 1989.

"When I refused an offer for a retirement party, two of my closest friends and colleagues came to my last class. With a great degree of humor, they told the class I was retiring but didn't want a party—so this was to take its place. They presented me with a power tool for my workshop. What they said and did meant far more than a dinner with many speeches. The bell rang and I retired."

"Do you consider your retirement to be an 'active' one?"

"Yes. I read a book in which the author differentiated between being busy and being active. A 'busy' person feels guilty when not busy or on the go doing something. The schedule and producing are still very important parts of life.

"The 'active' person has things to do but these can be mental and spiritual as well as physical. Time can be given to devotions, reading, sitting quietly to enjoy the scenery, rocking on the porch listening to birds singing with no feeling of guilt for not 'doing' or being productive. Few things have to be done 'right now' and even those few probably are not urgent.

"Since retiring my largest project is writing a book on family history for our four daughters and our grandchildren. Other projects include building a darkroom for black and white photography, telling stories to a class of six year olds taught by one of my former students, and working to keep the wooded area around the house a natural setting for wildlife. I can stop these activities to enjoy a colorful sunrise, a snowfall, or a rainbow with no feeling of guilt or pressure."

"Have you done volunteer work at your church?"

"Oh, yes. One great joy has been our church life—and the increase in my spiritual life. Peggy and I are active at New Providence Presbyterian Church in Maryville, Tennessee. Together, we have taught adult church school classes, worked on a Habitat for Humanity House project, and attended retreats. Each week I spend several hours studying scripture, reading writers such as C.S. Lewis, and meditating. I could have done this before retiring but never took the time.

"Three years ago I was asked if I would fill in for the pastor of visitation who was away for several weeks. I agreed and had a great time. When he decided not to return, I was asked to continue and now I visit about sixty members in retirement centers, in health centers, or shut-ins at home.

"I had heard 'You are more blessed when you visit than the people you visit' but never understood what was meant. Now I do. When I feel down, I visit Margery, ninety-nine years old and confined to bed. She greets me cheerfully and we have a fascinating conversation. I leave with my spirits lifted up. On these visits I have made some wonderful friends, have learned how people deal with adversity and pain, and have a better understanding of faith."

"Do you and your wife have similar retirement interests?

"Yes. Peggy retired two years ago and we do many things together. As I said, we work as a 'team' on several church activities. We like to cook so [we] spend time together in the kitchen preparing meals and trying new recipes. We are trying to hike to all of the waterfalls and cascades in the Smoky Mountain National Park. We are in an exercise program at the hospital, listen to music (classical, jazz of the forties), and walk in the nearby hills in the evening. And we enjoy talking to one another.

"We visit daughters in four different states as well as other family members, plan short trips in the region, and sometimes a two-week trip. Last year we returned to Heidelberg, Germany, where we met in 1947—when I was in the army and Peggy was in the U.S. dependent high school."

"Have you had to overcome any special problems in retirement?"

"No. We are now in excellent health. Last year, we talked to an insurance agent about a long-term health policy and he asked a number of health-related questions. One was 'Can you walk four blocks without getting out of breath?' We looked at each other and laughed. Two days earlier we made a strenuous fifteen-mile hike in the Smoky Mountains.

"Finances have not been a problem. We learned when I taught in public school and had two children, we could live on whatever we made. We took in free concerts, went on picnics instead of eating at restaurants, bought things on sale, did without, made or repaired things, and avoided buying on credit. We do the same now.

"I have two pet peeves about retirement attitudes. One is the cutesy signs on large RVs that say 'no job, no pay' or 'I'm spending my children's inheritance.' To some they may seem funny but they make retired people sound like whiners or selfish. The other peeve is the way older people are often portrayed in movies and on TV. How refreshing it would be to see a range of personalities in the media rather than stereotypes."

"What advice would you give a close friend about retirement?"

"Well," replied Bob, "My advice is: 'Begin planning before age fifty. Develop many interests. Have regular physical examinations. Have an exercise program in addition to any sports activity you may be in. Eat a heathful diet and eat small portions of food. Develop the ability to sit and relax for a time without TV being on or answering the telephone. And, if you are married, include your spouse in your planning—even though only one is retired, for both are involved.'

"As I said earlier, retirement is just another phase of life. I am enjoying it very much. It has been a positive experience and I am certain God has guided me along the way. Now, I want Peggy to have her say about retirement."

"Well, what are your thoughts on retirement?"

"I've heard it said that 'women's work' is never done. Some wives have complained, 'My retired husband is always underfoot and I can't get the housework done.' However, our retirement years have proved both those stereotypes to be false. Since I retired at sixty-two from the position of medical librarian at East Tennessee Children's Hospital, I've had many occasions to thank God that he led me to make the decision to join my husband in a very enjoyable and meaningful lifestyle.

"God's gift of time and energy to make our own choices is one of the greatest benefits of retirement. We have the freedom to invest that time and energy in a wide variety of activities. Recently I read a helpful statement by Oswald Chambers. He said, 'Spiritually, we never grow old; through the passing of the years we grow so many years *young*. . . The mature saint is just like a little child, absolutely simple and joyful and happy.' Bob and I have found this to be true as we spend more time with 'mature saints.'

"Did you feel that way at first?"

"Oh no. I remember the scary feeling of 'Now what do I do?' when our youngest daughter went away to college. I had concentrated on raising four daughters and being a full-time homemaker for so many years that the freedom to choose how to spend my time and energy was a gift I didn't know how to use. After talking it over with Bob, who was a great encourager, I went back to college and got a master's degree in education. I had been an elementary school teacher when we first married and thought I would go back to teaching. However, God had even better plans for me. Because I had been a volunteer in the hospital library, the librarian suggested I apply for her job when she resigned. It was the most interesting work I had ever done, and I was able to be of service to many doctors, nurses, and patients.

"When Bob retired, he became a volunteer at the hospital library and we worked as a team, not only at the library but also at home. He would have a delicious meal prepared on the days when he was at home and I was at work. We have continued to work together on many projects since I retired. For example, I enjoy making purses to sell at craft shows and he has designed signs and sales slips on the computer and helped in my booth. We also work as a team in church activities, home improvement projects, and family fun.

"We just had our 'almost' fifteen-year-old granddaughter spend ten days with us and had a great time sharing with her our love of hiking and dancing (she and I went to Jazzercise class together), and she went to church with us and helped serve refreshments at a circle meeting at our home. Bob especially enjoyed sharing family history with her, showing slides of her mother and her sisters when they were growing up and telling the story of how we met, grew to love each other, went to college together, married, and became a team that will have lasted fifty years in the year 2000.

"Bob has a story about a speaker who introduced his wife to his audience saying, 'We've had ten happy years together.' When his wife gasped in disbelief, he added, 'And out of forty years, that's not a bad average.' Bob and I both feel we've beat that average."

"*I admire the way you two help each other in retirement.*"

"Well, some of our best preparation for retirement has been at times when we had to be very flexible about gender roles. For example, just before he retired, Bob had colon surgery. He had always been the 'take charge' leader in our family, but while he was recuperating in the hospital, I found temporary housing for us to live in while our new retirement home, 'Simple Gifts,' was being built. 'Take Charge Bob' was forced to sit and watch while our Sunday school class, daughter, son-in-law, and I moved us out of the home we'd lived in for twenty-five years.

"It was a valuable learning experience for all of us. He had asked me when I was going through the empty-nest syndrome if I'd like to switch places with him. Since then, we've discovered that we switch places back and forth all the time—and it makes life much more fun."

"*Has anyone served as a retirement role model for you?*"

"Oh yes. Just as children and adolescents need models and mentors, I think retirees do, too. Bob mentioned the ones he sees as he visits for the church. I have a great example in my eighty-eight-year-old father who retired from the army after twenty years of service. He has been playing tournament tennis, serving his church, and traveling with 'Friendship Force' and elderhostel programs ever since. I hope that Bob and I can serve in the same capacity for our children and grandchildren."

Sharing Stage and Screen Skills with Twentieth-Century Adventurers

PHYLLIS LOVE "OSANNA" GOODING

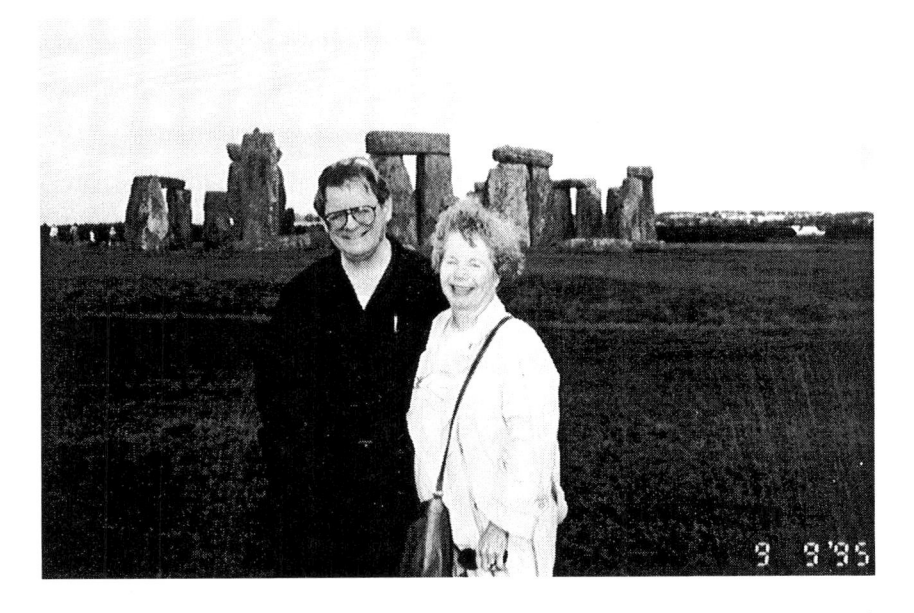

"What did you do before retirement?" I asked retired stage and screen actress Phyllis Love "Osanna" Gooding.

"Well, my life falls into three distinct careers, actually, as I view it now at age seventy. In my twenties and thirties, after majoring in theatre and graduating from Carnegie Institute of Technology, I was a professional actress—fortunate enough to have played the ingenue of eight original Broadway productions. Three of those were by some of our most famous playwrights: *The Country Girl* by Clifford Odets, *The Rose Tattoo* by Tennessee Williams, and *Bus Stop* by William Inge.

"During this period I also starred in numerous TV shows and acted in two movies: *The Young Doctors* and *Friendly Persuasion*, in which I played the Quaker daughter of Gary Cooper and Dorothy McGuire. My stage name was Phyllis Love."

"What was the second career?"

"My second career began in a Southern California high school where I taught English and some drama for fifteen years. Teaching proved as dramatic as show business for our school in the early 1970s became integrated and, along with the community, strove to become a model for the nation. Our white students, in the main, were looking forward to integration and befriended the early black students, and vice-versa, but the administration made a disastrous mistake. Minority students from the Los Angeles tough inner city were allowed to register in our suburban school with phoney addresses, instead of the rigorous use of utility bills and other validation required now. Some of the out-of-town youths pulled knives and extorted lunch money from the white students right on campus. This initiated rapid white flight and the death of our dream of a harmoniously integrated school and community.

"In my private life my first husband, a playwright and a poet, became mentally ill in 1959. That condition improved enough by 1977 so that he could support himself as a nighttime security guard at Bob Hope's Touluca Lake estate. His job allowed me to follow my inner receiving that God had found me faithful and now I was free. We divorced that fall." Osanna's expressive voice and face were animated as she shared her story.

"What was that third career you mentioned?"

"My third career began in my fifty-sixth year, in 1982. Shakespeare says 'ripeness is all.' I say ripeness and timing are all and appear to me, and to Alan Gooding, my second husband, able to effect a seeming miracle. He, an attorney, and I crossed paths in the Los Angeles County Courthouse and he recognized me after not seeing me for twenty-seven years. At that long-ago-time, he had come backstage to see me in my Broadway dressing room after attending my current play *The Remarkable Mr. Penneypacker*.

"Years before that we had been engaged college sweethearts before I had gone off to act in summer stock in the East—and had met the visiting older playwright who soon became my first husband.

Six months after our courthouse reunion, I retired from teaching and married my best friend and soulmate. This third career fulfilled a deep life-long hole in my heart. I became an instant stepmother to four wonderful live-in children, ages seven to fourteen."

"When did you become leader of the Writers' Group for retirees at Westminster Gardens?"

"Oh, that favorite retirement project began in 1986, overlapping with my stepmothering opportunity. Upon submission of my co-authored film script, *The Seventh Trouble*, to the California Endowment of the Arts Council, I was given a grant to establish a Writers' Group for retired Presbyterian missionaries and other church workers in their Westminster Gardens retirement community in Duarte, California. The grant ended in a year, but ten years later I'm still there. From January through May each year, I serve as the convener and leader of this fascinating group of old and new members—sharing and giving critical feedback on their varied writings. These include memoirs, plays, poetry, articles, essays, meditations, letters to the editor, short stories, science fiction, fairy tales, and historical accounts of a time we shall not see again."

"Please share your impressions regarding the group."

"They are productive people. About eleven of them have had mission stories published by the Celebrate Curriculum of the Presbyterian (U.S.A.) Church. Two have had articles published in the magazine *Presbyterians Today*, and one has had an article published in the Baptist magazine *Home Life* and in the Baptist magazine for boys called *Pioneer*. One has had two articles published in the Presbyterian magazine *Monday Morning*. Several are writing books and one has managed to publish six books since 1992, with a seventh one due out in October, 1997.

"As I think about the group, past images fast-forward and flood my mind. . . tall, slim, white-haired Harry Dorman, a fifth-generation American missionary teacher serving in Lebanon, during a reading of his play *Come Home, Come Home* in Packard Hall in front of all the Westminster Gardens residents. Harry, after Paul Robeson and Dylan Thomas, had the most magnificent speaking voice I've ever heard. As he read the part of the old Lebanese patriarch Abu-Hassan, he transformed that lectern into a rugged cliff overlooking crashing, pounding surf below as he howled

'Ammar,' 'Hassan,' 'Ammar,' 'Hassan,'—the names of his farmer sons who had sailed to visit 1920s, party-time, speakeasy America and who had not written or returned . . ." With a far away look in her eyes, Osanna continued her images.

"Edith Moser, age ninety, complex, depreciating her own writing skill, despite our multiple coaxing—one day gleefully bursting into our meeting waving in the air her unforgettable memoir titled *Chickens*. Edith described hand-carrying Rhode Island Red chicken eggs, purchased in Sao Paulo on the coast, back to their school and farm station in the isolated Mato Grosso interior of Brazil. She had high hopes of improving the native breed of scrawny, tasteless chickens. She wrote 'First there were five days on a wobbly narrow gage train, transfer to a twenty-four-hour boat, wait four days in a hotel to get a small river boat to take my husband and me up the river for eight days—then a day of eight hours on horseback to our farm.'

"This remarkable woman and her agronomist husband were on their own in this wilderness for years. The promised preacher and teacher never arrived. Edith grew a large vegetable garden to feed their Indian students and her family. She sewed clothes and cooked for all. She taught school and Bible study. She played piano and directed the choir and somehow taught the children to play five different instruments that she'd never played herself.

"Edith was one of the ones who, through action, defined for me the reality of a *sincere* Christian. One of her students was Augusto, the son of a chief of the Nambequare Indians who had massacred five American missionaries stationed in Central America. After two years at their school, Augusto went home carrying under his arm his very own Rhode Island Red rooster and a love for Jesus. . . ." Her eyes sparkling with excitement, Osanna continued.

"A more cosmopolitan setting—Bangkok, Thailand. Mary Chaffee and her pastor-teacher husband Cliff rent a nice house and are helping develop a church and a church school. Mary mainly taught music at the school and, later, throughout the city—as she produced and sang in and conducted opera music, becoming known throughout Bangkok as 'Mrs. Music.' A different setting here for evangelizing but the same rock-bottom salaries, and the 'stuff' of life— clothes, blankets, toys—were much needed and periodically arrived in their sponsors churches' large charity box of parishioners' cast-

Sharing Stage and Screen Skills with Twentieth-Century Adventurers 157

offs. But financial facts could never influence Mary to condone an action that seemed wrong to her.

"Her Chinese cook, Tian, announced one day that he and his wife could not feed their expected fifth child and so they were going to sell the new baby.

"Mary cried, 'No, you must not sell the baby!' The cook shouted back that his salary and his wife's laundry payments just barely paid for themselves and their four children.

"Again Mary fought, 'If you sell the baby, you leave! God gave you and Etai this precious baby. You cannot give it away.'

"Cook Tian snapped back, 'Then you take the baby. You raise the baby. The baby will be yours!'

"Mary suddenly knew the answer. She explained to Cook Tian that they had a very small income and she, herself, was expecting another child. 'All that my baby has I can share with you. My child's food will be your child's food. Diapers, clothing, blankets, vitamins, toys, medical care—we will give to your baby the same as we give to our own baby.'

"The two baby girls became and remain lifelong friends, both were educated, and both are fluent in Thai and in English.

"*You mean your horizons were broadened by contact with missionaries like Harry, Edith, and Mary?*"

"Oh, yes. Working with these intelligent, highly educated Christians has given me enormous gifts—not book knowledge, but the knowledge of the history in my lifetime of ordinary people around the globe as they lived it, and that understanding has helped me to grasp the concept of 'one mankind.' There are so many fascinating glimpses of different cultures—I feel that five months of every year for the last decade I've been on a round-the-world tour.

"Too many scenes to enumerate, but running through my mind this day...Stan Wick (I and my whole family are on his daily prayer list of hundreds of people) venturing into the toughest bars in Guatemala to tell the habitues how Jesus loves them. His Quiche Indian parishioner returning peace and friendship to the powerful witch doctors who opposed and abused them—winning some of those enemies over to their faith. . .

"Another image: Preacher Donald Reasoner, with a one thousand square mile parish in Brazil whose new parishioners were so strong in their faith they were able to exorcise a demon from a mother and housewife. She had been possessed for six years by a foul-mouthed demon named 'Satan' who continually threw the food she had fixed for her family on the floor—while cursing them out in a voice other than her own...

"The image of Dr. Frank Newman and nurse wife Betty serving in China, doctoring the hundreds of Chinese the Japanese frequently bombed in World War II. Then they returned after the war to a China overrun by the Communists in 1949. They stayed on. But one and a-half years later, after many house inspections, office interrogations, and house arrest, they were finally tried as foreign spies in a 'peoples court.' They were 'convicted' of being 'foreign devil American spies.' Their fellow Chinese Christians saved their lives by outshouting the government stooges who had been instructed to pronounce a death sentence. To save them, their friends shouted 'kick the foreign devils out of China!' drowning out the stooges' 'Execute them!'

"Moving to Cameroon, Africa, Dr. Newman invented a new technique for treating elephantiasis. Instead of cutting off the thickened, leathery, huge, ulcerated, and stinking lower legs of the patients, he cut two- by six-inch skin grafts from the normal upper legs and sewed them together. Then he cut off all the diseased skin from the lower legs and wrapped the healthy skin around them like a stocking—protected with antibiotics, in two weeks, a new leg!

"Frank also may have been the first doctor in the world to take the patients' own blood before an operation, store it in a refrigerator, and then transfuse it back into the patient after the operation. Now, with AIDS and other diseases, this is a common practice."

"As one who has benefitted from your guidance to the Writers' Group, I am deeply grateful for your kind encouragement and help. How would you summarize your experience with the group?"

"Well, at first I feared there would be a lot of pious words and prayers from the group. Instead I got to know trained workers who were actively trying to live the teachings of Christ. I found that, in the main, it was the downtrodden poor, the politically oppressed, the medically neglected, and the educationally deprived who had been served by these great adventurers of the twentieth century.

"These teachers, preachers, doctors, and nurses at home and in Asia, South America, Africa, and the Middle East wanted to share God's love for humanity with people from all walks of life. And they are still at it. Knowing these retirees, my fear of old age has evaporated. These 'retired' folks continue to learn, to help others in their own and surrounding communities.

"To the joy of my soul these retired seventy-, eighty-, and ninety-year-olds, despite some aches and pains, are still the joyful servants of the Lord."

Insights Gained from These Retirees

What can we learn from these retirees? They deal with several issues relating to making retirement meaningful and enjoyable. One retiree points out the wisdom of planning ahead for retirement. She says, "I invested in a tax-free IRA (Individual Retirement Account) plus other investments. She adds, "Most of all prepare yourself mentally and spiritually. I did, and I am enjoying every minute of my retirement."

Another retiree said, "I began planning for retirement years before the event." A third retiree said, "My wife and I thought carefully about what kind of retirement location we wanted. . . . We wanted a place where we had educational stimulation. . . . We also wished for good medical facilities. . . . We desired cultural opportunities. . . but most of all we sought a good church life for spiritual stimulation." He adds that they planned ahead and found these things at Maryville, Tennessee, where he had once taught at Maryville College—early in his teaching career.

Several retirees implied a direct relationship between how well they planned for retirement and how happy, and satisfied, they are with their retirement situation.

I live in a retirement community of over two hundred retirees. Most planned well for their retirement, but a few did not. It is obvious that those who planned well have fewer problems than those who did not plan.

Most of the retirees I interviewed seem to value volunteer work and participate in some type of volunteer service. The places of service include nursing homes, hospitals, libraries, and schools—in addition to volunteer work for family and friends. At a YWCA meeting honoring one retiree volunteer, she was given credit for volunteer work with eleven different groups.

One retiree volunteer tells of her work in a library, hospital, nursing home, and two churches. But perhaps the most active retiree volunteer was one who retired in Nashville, Tennessee. She did work with a group called "Peace Links" (working for world peace). She did "Telephone Helpline" work with the Crisis Center there. She did work with the American Association of University Women, Church Women United, Interfaith Community Outreach (helping needy people), and the YWCA (teaching English to foreign students and immigrants), and she led a Canasta Club at her local Senior Center.

Having done volunteer visiting in nursing homes and hospitals myself, I can understand how meaningful such volunteer work became for these retirees. However, my greatest admiration goes to those retirees who did volunteer work that is perhaps even more difficult and demanding. Several worked in centers providing food, clothing, and shelter for needy people. Another helped to rehabilitate prostitutes; one became the main leader in helping a group of women to start a shelter for battered women.

All of these retiree volunteers seem to imply that they do volunteer work not only to serve others but also because the volunteer work enriches their own life. It makes them feel useful and fulfilled. And I am amazed at how many different types of volunteer work these retirees found to do. That has convinced me that, in our retirement, each one of us can find some type of volunteer service that is appropriate for us.

One retiree makes the point that retirement should include new activities. He says, "For me that means enjoying reading, listening to music, hiking, photography, storytelling, searching family history and photos, writing and working in the yard—especially being active in my church and enjoying time with family."

He makes a distinction between being "active" and being busy." He says, "A 'busy' person feels guilty when not busy or on the go doing something. . . the 'active' person has things to do but these can be mental and spiritual as well as physical. Time can be given to devotions, reading, sitting quietly to enjoy the scenery, rocking on the porch and listening to birds singing with no feeling of guilt for not 'doing' or being productive."

Another says, "I have more choices for reading, research, writing. . . . I can begin gardening when the weather permits, not when I have caught up on my paper grading."

A third retiree said, "About five years ago I pursued a 'dream' that I had—which was to play the piano for entertainment purposes at some place where people mingled, such as a cruise ship or a shopping mall. . . . I began playing three-hour sessions at Arcadia Mall."

New activities in retirement are important, but using special skills from preretirement work should also be considered. I have two retired friends who are medical doctors. Both have done very helpful volunteer work in hospitals in India and in Africa.

Continuing education seems to be a goal for many of these retirees. Several said how much they enjoy going to Elderhostels—where education, sightseeing, and recreation are all included in one financially reasonable package. One couple said that in twelve years they have attended twenty-three Elderhostels in six states—stretching from California to Virginia.

One retiree tells of taking continuing education courses in a college and a university. Another tells of taking creative writing classes and learning to sing—even learning to sing solos. He also learned to adjust to a new bride at age eighty-eight—when he married a young woman of seventy-seven. Learning new things and doing new things can add real spice to life.

Recreation and exercise became more appealing and possible for some of these retirees, after gaining more free time in retirement. One retiree tells about playing golf three times a week with friends—beginning at 6:30 a.m. He adds that he also does active jobs around the house that increase his exercise opportunities. Another tells of daily walks with her husband and their dog, enjoying the beautiful sunrises. After giving up golf due to a bad back, one woman walks with a friend every weekday morning for half an hour.

Exercising with others makes it easier and also brings the added benefit of fellowship and fun. Among the two hundred-plus retirees in my retirement community, about fifteen are still able to play tennis. One said, "When playing tennis, I am having so much fun and fellowship I don't even realize I am exercising." One here still plays tennis at age eighty-seven and another at age ninety-two. Even after receiving a heart "pacemaker" at age seventy-six, I was later able to return to tennis. None of us here will ever be a Pete Sampras, but we do have fun, fellowship, and good exercise.

Several retirees emphasized the importance of having good personal relationships in retirement. One tells how she and her husband learned to work as a "team" in retirement. This meant becoming "flexible" about changing gender roles in taking care of household tasks and other duties. Another says, "My helping to lighten my wife's household burdens doesn't mean taking over her world, but it does mean sharing her burdens in a helpful way." A third retiree said personal relationships were the "bottom line" of a lifetime of ministry with his wife—as they worked with many wonderful people.

One of the so-called "intangible" factors that can help to make retirement meaningful and enjoyable is humor. One retiree sees the humor of the situation when a retirement job selling real estate makes him the "token male" in an office dominated by fourteen women. He joked with me that he never had to accuse any of them of "sexual harassment" toward him. Another retiree sees humor in celebrating his eighty-three birthdays on "income tax day." He says that his birthday being on income tax day has enabled his wife to remember his birthday every year for fifty-three years of married life together. A third retiree jokes that one good thing about being too busy in retirement is that "God, family, friends, and activities are enough to keep us out of mischief."

I especially like the ability of one retiree to laugh at himself—even regarding humorous situations caused by his health problems. He says, "It sends my wife into gales of laughter every time I tell her I am having a 'hot flash'" (due to female hormones he has to take for prostate cancer treatments). He adds, "My wife also kids me because the medicine I take makes me put on weight. . . . because I have told her in the past that my trim figure was due to 'right thoughts and clean living.'"

Several retirees indicate that their faith in God to guide and help them, when they face a crisis in retirement, has proven to be an invaluable asset. When she lost her husband, one retiree said, "I soon discovered that, although my friends and family can help, ultimately I had to work out my grief with God." After her son took his own life, another retiree said, ". . . all I could say was God please help us. . . give us the strength to go on living. . . repeating the words of the twenty-third Psalm 'though I walk through the valley of the shadow of death, Thou art with me.'" Almost all of these retirees indicate that faith in God helps them face aging and retirement problems. I can see that it helps them to endure many aches and pains with amazingly little complaining.

Having to care for his Alzheimer's wife twenty-four hours a day, one retiree says, ". . . I am learning that Christ is giving me a new calling . . . the call of God to the *vocation* of caring for my wife. . . I am learning that Christ himself identifies with me . . . since Christ is with me day by day I shouldn't worry. . . . Christ is teaching me patience. . . . Another comforting Bible verse promise is 'As your days, so shall your strength be'" (Deut. 33:25).

Now let's sum up some of the insights we have gained from these retirees, and try to draw some conclusions from these insights. We must not try to conclude too much. However, I do think it is safe to say that these insights indicate that a meaningful and enjoyable retirement should include the following elements: early planning for retirement; volunteer work that not only serves others but also brings a feeling of usefulness and fulfillment to the volunteer; appropriate housing, with pleasant surroundings; choosing helpful exercise and recreational activities; good health care for present and future needs; learning new things and doing new things; learning the difference between being meaningfully "active" versus merely being "busy" (including knowing the difference between "doing" and "being"); maintaining good relationships, especially having married couples act as a cooperative "team" (being flexible about traditional gender roles); having a positive attitude toward retirement; keeping a good sense of humor; and having faith in God to guide and help when facing a crisis, such as serious illness or losing a loved one.

I am impressed by the important role that so-called "intangible" values seem to play in the life of many of these retirees. Some examples are the following: the overall positive attitude toward retirement that most of them demonstrate; the importance of maintaining a sense of humor in retirement; and especially the value many seem to see in having faith that God will guide and help them through difficult times.

I think the overall conclusion for us from these retirees is that, if we act on the insights they have shared with us, most of us can have a retirement that is indeed meaningful and enjoyable. However, there are some important issues that they do not deal with in depth. One is the issue of loneliness faced by some retirees, both women and men.

One retiree briefly addresses this, saying she alleviates her loneliness by seeking meaningful relationships with "cousins by the dozens" and with her "church family". But she does something else that almost any lonely single retiree can do. She joined service groups, such as the "Senior Singers" she mentions. Like her, other lonely retirees can join some service group and bring joy to others and at the same time overcome their loneliness by finding meaningful new relationships. One of the good examples shown by these retirees is the group called "The Good Eggs," who join together to drive lonely people to doctors and dentists, feed the hungry, and take lonely people out to lunch.

A wise person said, "God loves us just the way we are, but God loves us too much to leave us the way we are." I believe God wants to help lonely singles to find meaningful relationships that help all persons involved. It takes both a "family" and a "village" to meet all retirees' needs.

Since these retirees are still reasonably healthy and active, another issue they do not deal with here (but may need to address later) is the problem of catastrophic illness. For those with adequate financial resources, a catastrophic illness insurance plan is possible. However, for those without adequate resources for private insurance plans, a larger group plan should be considered. Some health specialists seem to think that this may eventually need to be worked out on a state or national level.

Government statistics indicate that senior citizens are the fastest growing segment of our society. (See the appendix.) Therefore, there is an urgent need to learn how to deal with all the issues related to aging and retirement.

Appendix:
Graphs of Age Groups in the U.S.A.
(from 1900 to 2030)

U.S. Population by Age and Sex, 1900, 1970, 1995, and 2030

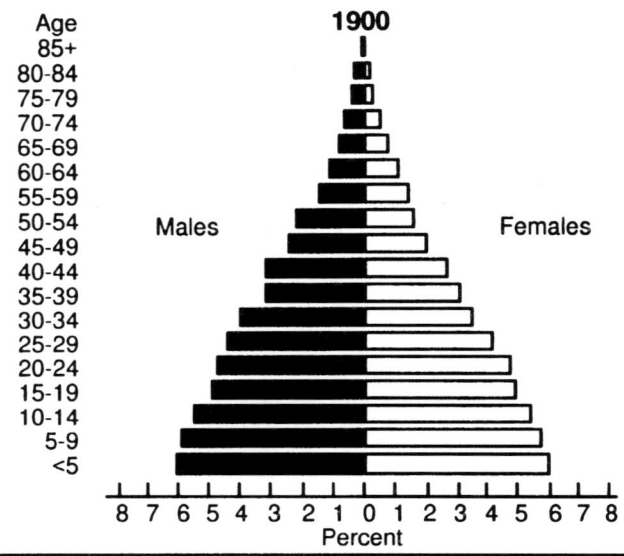

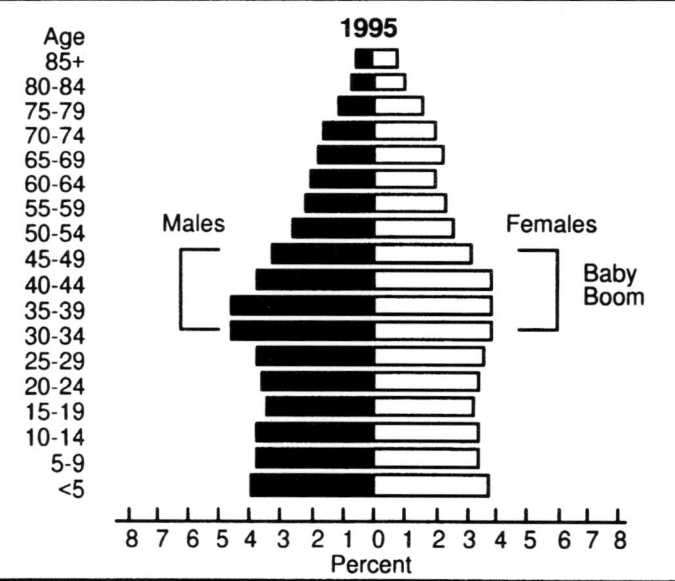

1900

1995 — Baby Boom (ages 30-34 to 45-49)

1970

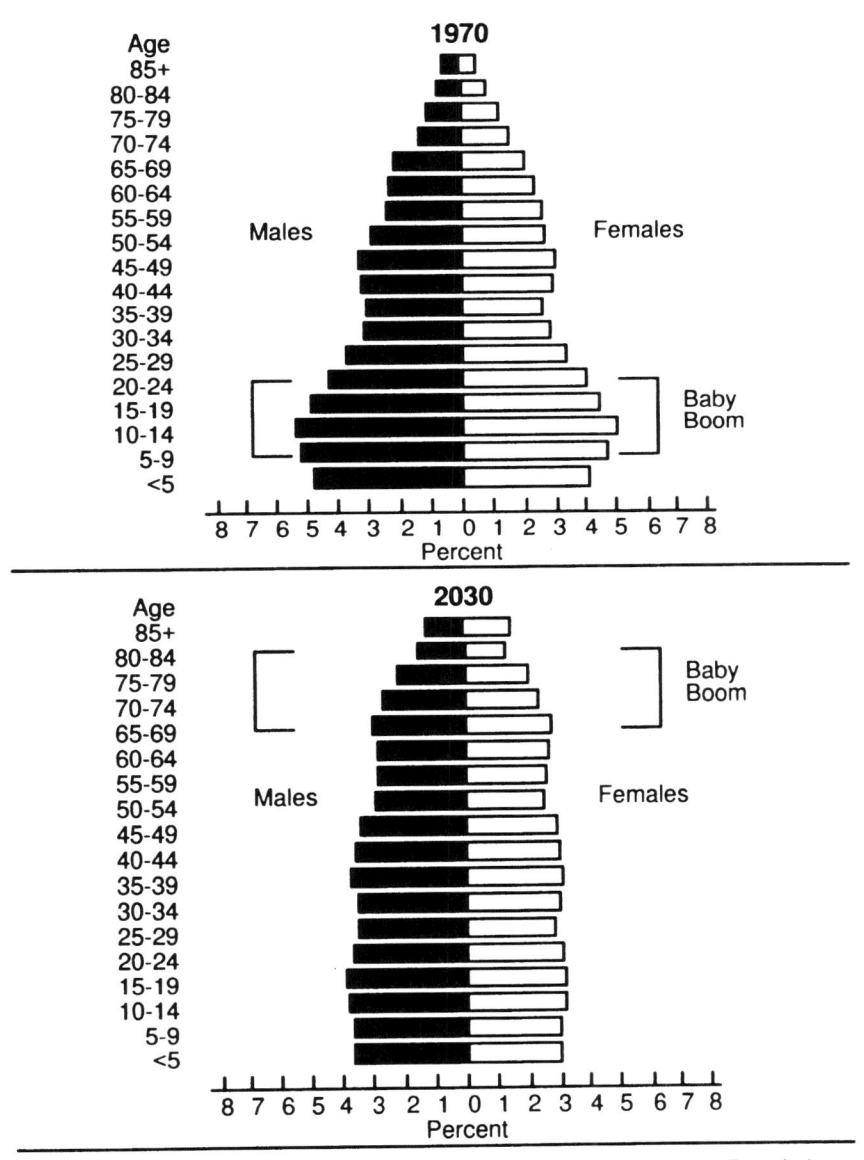

Age	Males	Females
85+		
80-84		
75-79		
70-74		
65-69		
60-64		
55-59		
50-54		
45-49		
40-44		
35-39		
30-34		
25-29		
20-24		Baby Boom
15-19		
10-14		
5-9		
<5		

Percent: 8 7 6 5 4 3 2 1 0 1 2 3 4 5 6 7 8

2030

Age	Males	Females
85+		
80-84		Baby Boom
75-79		
70-74		
65-69		
60-64		
55-59		
50-54		
45-49		
40-44		
35-39		
30-34		
25-29		
20-24		
15-19		
10-14		
5-9		
<5		

Percent: 8 7 6 5 4 3 2 1 0 1 2 3 4 5 6 7 8

Treas, J. (1995). "Older Americans in the 1990s and Beyond." In *Populations Bulletin, 50*. Washington, DC: Population Reference Bureau, Inc.

Glossary

Alcoholics Anonymous: A support group to help alcoholic persons.

Alzheimer's disease: A form of senility with mental confusion.

atrial fibrillation: Fast, irregular heartbeat.

AAUW: American Association of University Women.

battered women: Women abused by husband or boyfriend.

bush hog: A machine for cutting down weeds and bushes.

code blue: Hospital code for a heart attack.

crib death: Unexpected death of infants in their cribs.

CWU: Church Women United.

elderhostel: A study program for older people, including recreation.

elephantiasis: Enormous enlargement of a body part, usually by filarial worms.

enabler: One who helps others to get things done.

genealogy: A record or study of family history.

general conference: Ruling body of a national church, as Methodists, Holiness, etc.

guinea fowl: An African bird related to the pheasant, raised for eggs and meat.

halfway house: A home to help troubled people get back into society.

idiom: A particular language or dialect, an expression peculiar to a speaking style.

interim pastor: A temporary fill-in minister of a church.

internment camp: A camp used to intern Japanese in America in World War II.

locum: A temporary fill-in pastor for a Presbyterian church in New Zealand.

polymyalgia rheumatica: A type of autoimmune disease, causing painful muscles.

Presbyterian and Reformed Church terms:

   elder: Officer in a local church ruling body.

   General Assembly: Highest ruling body, made up of elected ministers, elders.

   moderator: Presiding officer of a ruling body.

   presbytery: Organized group of local churches, made up of ministers and elder representatives who form the ruling body for those churches.

   session: Ruling body of a local church, active elders with minister as moderator.

   synod: Ruling body for an organized group of presbyteries.

RV: recreational vehicle.

Scots/Welsh games: A sports program for ethnic Scots and Welsh people.

tamoxifen: A type of chemotherapy medication for cancer.

Tentmaker: A Christian evangelist who supports his/her work with a secular job, like the Apostle Paul making tents in biblical days.

Bibliography

Boyd, M. (1996). "Look Outward for New Directions." *Modern Maturity*, May-June 1996, p.79.

Chappell, N. (1990). "Aging and Social Care." In R. Binstock, and L. George (eds.), *The Handbook of Aging and the Social Sciences*. San Diego, CA: Academic Press.

Clements, W. (ed.) (1989). *Ministry with the Aging*. Binghamton, NY: The Haworth Press, Inc.

Clements, W. (ed.) (1989). *Religion, Aging, and Health*. Binghamton, NY: The Haworth Press, Inc.

Conrad, W. R., and Glenn, W. R. (1976). *The Effective Voluntary Board of Directors*. Chicago, IL: The Swallow Press.

Cooper, C. (1976). "Swimming for Senior Citizens." *Therapeutic Recreation Journal*, 2, pp. 50-54.

Crimmins, E., and D. Ingegneri. (1990). "Interaction and Living Arrangements of Older Parents and Their Children: Past Trends, Present Determinants, Future Implications." *Research on Aging*, 12(1), pp. 3-33.

Dye, H. *The Touch of Friendship: Broadening Social Relationships in the Senior Years*. Nashville, TN: Baptist Sunday School Board.

Goldman, C., and R. Mahler. (1995). *Secrets of Becoming a Late Bloomer: Extraordinary Ordinary People on the Art of Staying Creative, Active, and Aware in Mid-Life and Beyond*. Walpole, NH: Stillpoint Publishing.

Hendrickson, M. (ed.) (1986). *The Role of the Church in Aging*, Volumes I, II, III. Binghamton, NY: The Haworth Press, Inc.

Iacocca, L. (1996). "I Flunked Retirement." *Fortune*, June 24, p. 50 ff.

Jernigan, H., with M. Jernigan (1992). *Aging in Chinese Society: A Holistic Approach to the Experience of Aging in Taiwan and Singapore*. Binghamton, NY: The Haworth Press, Inc.

Jorgensen, J. (1980). *The Graying of America: Retirement and Why You Can't Afford It*. New York: McGraw-Hill Paperbacks.

Koenig, H. (1994). *Aging and God: Spiritual Pathways to Mental Health in Mid-life and Later Years*. Binghamton, NY: The Haworth Pastoral Press.

Lewis, R. (1995). "Creative Time Looming Ahead." *AARP Bulletin*, January 1995, 36(1), p. 2.

Morgan, R. (1993). *I Never Found That Rocking Chair: God's Call at Retirement*. Nashville, TN: Upper Room Books.

Palder, E. (1989). *The Retirement Sourcebook*. Kensington, MD: Woodbine House.

Robb, T. (1991) *Growing Up: Pastoral Nurture for the Later Years*. Binghamton, NY: The Haworth Pastoral Press.

Rosow, I. (1967). *Social Integration of the Aged*. New York: Free Press.

Seeber, J. (ed.) (1991). *Spiritual Maturity in the Later Years*. Binghamton, NY: The Haworth Pastoral Press.

Sessoms, B. *Ideas for Activities with Senior Adults*. Nashville, TN: Baptist Sunday School Board.

Treas, J. (1995). "Older Americans in the 1990s and Beyond." *Populations Bulletin*, 50. Washington, DC: Population Reference Bureau, Inc.

Uris, A. (1979). *Over 50: The Definitive Guide to Retirement*. Radnor, PA: Chilton Book Co.

Webber, A. (1990). *Life Later On: Older People and the Church*. London: Triangle.

Willcocks, I., S. Peace, and L. Keller. (1986). *Private Lives in Public Places*. London: Tavistock Press.

Index

Acting, 153-154
"Active" vs. "busy," 148-149,162
Advice. *See* Planning
African clinic, 5
AIDS, 55
Alaska, 70,76
Alzheimer's disease, 1,7-10,65-67, 165
American Association of University Women, 17,24-25
Art and craftwork, 54
Asthma, 54-55
Attitudes in retirement, 150
Audiovisual program, 61-64

Baptism, 124
Beanland, Gayle, 61-64
Bible study, 59,102,119
Birds, feeding, 65-66,111
Blind, recording books on tape for, 28-29
Book fair, 23-24
Books on tape, 28-29
Bread for the World, 17
Breast cancer, 101,103-104
Brown, Mildred (Millie), 99-104
Bushing, Arthur, 57-60
"Busy" vs. "active," 148-149, 162-163

Caldwell, Robert L., 95-98
Cancer, 101,103-104
Car accident, 79
Caregiving
  for aging parents, 113
  for extended family, 125

Caregiving *(continued)*
  grandparents in, 12
  for son, 54-55
  for spouse
    with Alzheimer's, 1,7-10,54-55, 65-67,165
  marriage and, 133
Catastrophic illness, 166
Celebrations, 78-79
Chambers, Oswald, 151
Chickens (Moser), 156
Child care centers, 42
Children. *See* Family
Christian giving training, 35-38
Chronicles of Narnia (Lewis), 128
Church. *See also* Spirituality
  Bible study, 59
  Christian giving training, 35-38
  evangelization, 144,145-146
  pastors, 52-53
    interim, 95-98,107,138
    in New Zealand, 76-77,97-98
    in Santa Cruz, 52-53
    visitation and counseling, 76
    on Yavapai-Apache Indian Reservation, 71-72
  serving in Japan in retirement, 115-117
  visitation and transportation, 82-84
  volunteering in,12-13,18,19,24, 32-33,41-42,44-45,92,111, 119,145
    administration, 134-135
    editing newsletter, 134
    visitation, 149
  women's organizations, 124-125

175

Church Women United, 18
Colossians 1:11, 10
Come Home, Come Home (Dorman), 155
Community service, 23,24,92,93. *See also* Volunteering
  in elementary schools, 29
Computers, 140
Consulting work, 110
Continuing education, 106
  Elderhostel, 13,23
  genealogy, 12
  importance of, 163
  new activities, 1
II Corinthians 10:4,5, 146
II Corinthians 12:8, 144
Counseling, 76
Cultural issues. *See* Multicultural issues
Cultural opportunities, 106

Dandelion, 129
Davis, Hal and Kirby, 43-46
Death/dying, 42. *See also* Grieving
Demographics, 1
Deuteronomy 33:25, 10,165
Diet, 27-28,84
Disabilities, 138
Dorman, Harry, 155
Douthitt, Jim, 69-73

Economic planning, 1,25
Editing newsletter, 103,134
Education. *See* Continuing education
Elderhostel, 13,23,119,163
Employment
  reducing responsibilities, 58-59
  in retirement
    consulting, 110
    farming, 91-92
    in Japan, 115-117
    as pastors, 52,95-98,107,138
    real estate sales, 97
    teaching, 17,91,101-103,135

Engelhardt, Leroy (Roy), 105-108
English as a Second Language, 17, 101-102,135
Entertaining, international students, 112-113
Ethiopia, 37
Evangelization, 144,145-146
Exercise and recreation, 19,42,50, 110-111
  "active" vs. "busy," 148-149
  advice for, 60
  cultural opportunities, 106
  golf, 12,84
  health and, 89,119,140
  importance of, 162-163
  similar interests, 149-150
  tennis, 73
  walking, 12

Fair housing laws, 72
Faith. *See* Church; Spirituality
Family, 40. *See also* Marriage
  caregiving for, 12,44,54-55,113, 125
  death of son, 55,120-121
  grandchildren, 66-67,152
  proximity, 118-119
  relationship with parents, 117-118
  as support, 126-127
  travel to visit, 139-140
Farming, 91-93
Finances, 150
Financial planning, 25
Finch, Nelly, 91-93
First Fruits (Lindholm), 37
First Things First (Gray), 53
Food banks, 41
Friendships. *See* Personal relationships
Furgerson, Helen, 109-113

Gardening, 40,110,140
Gender roles, 108,152
Genealogy, 12

Golf, 12,84
Gooding, Phyllis Love "Osanna," 153-159
Gordon-Conwell Theological Seminary, 144-145
Grandparents, caregiving, 12
Gray, Joe, 51-55
Grieving, 49
   death of son, 55,120-121
   loneliness, 93
   relocation and, 93
   spirituality and, 164-165
   support groups, 93
   volunteering in healing, 11-12

Habitat for Humanity, 34
Hansen, June, 31-34
Harvey, Earle, 75-80
Hawaii, 69-70
Health, 19,42,50,59-60,150. *See also* Caregiving
   breast cancer, 101,103-104
   catastrophic illness, 166
   disabilities, 138
   eating habits, 27-28,84
   exercise and, 119,140
   heart disease, 79,89
   helping others and, 45-46
   holistic approach, 111-112
   humor and, 164
   medication side effects, 45
   polymyalgia rheumatica, 77
   retirement and, 93
   shingles, 125-126
   spirituality and, 144
   stomach cancer, 131-132
   volunteering and, 33-34
Heart disease, 79,89
Hereford, Nannie, 15-19
Hobbies. *See* Exercise and recreation; *specific activities*
Homeless people, 33
Horcher, Dot, 123-129

Hospital chaplaincy, 86-87
Hospitality, international students, 112-113
Hospitals, volunteering, 23
Housewives, 123
Housing, 22,107,110
Hoyt, Mary Ruth, 1,21-25
Humor, 81,88-89,164
   nursing home residents, 5

Immigration, 72,101-102,138-139
Interim pastors, 52,95-98,107,138
International students, 112-113
InterVarsity Missionaries Convention, 146
Iranians, 72-73
Isaiah 40:31, 121
Iyoya, Rhoda, 2,115-121

Jamison, Eleanor, 1,11
Jamison, Frank, 81-84
Japan, 29
   missionaries to, 15-16
   retirement in, 101
   serving U.S. service personnel and families in, 115-117
   teaching in, 99-100,103-104
Japanese-American internment, 137-138
Japanese students, 102,135

Lazear, Bob, 1,7-10
Learning. *See* Continuing education
Lewis, C. S., 128
Library volunteer work, 22-23
Lindholm, Paul, 35
Literacy teaching, 103
Loneliness, 93,166
Lowe, Henry (Tim), 65-67

McClelland Johnson, Vicki, 2,47-50
McIntire, Bob, 61-64

Mackenzie, Virginia, 2,27-30
Marriage, 47-50,124
　adjustments in retirement, 108, 132,152
　caregiving of spouse, 1,7-10, 54-55,65-67,133,165
　remarriage, 50,55
　renewal of vows, 133-134
　similar interests in retirement, 149-150
　volunteering as team, 151-152
　wedding anniversary, 78-79
Mary Magdalene Project, 40-41
Maryville, Tennessee, 106-107,149
Maryville College, 47-48,57-58
Matthew 6:21, 37
Matthew 6:33, 84
Matthew 6:34, 10,121
Matthew 11:28-30, 9
Medication, side effects, 45
Memory, 30
Mental illness, 55
Mentors, 58
Missionaries, 155-159.
　See also Church
　to Japan, 15-16
Monte Vista Grove retirement community, 118-119
More To Be Desired Than Gold (Wilson), 145
Moser, Edith, 156
Multicultural issues
　Christian giving training, 35-38
　Japanese, 102-103,116-117
Music, 53-54,64,77-78,106
Muslims, 145-146
Mutability, 60

Nashville, 16-18
Navajo Indians, 71
Navajo Sunrise (Gray), 51-52,53
New Zealand, 76-77,97-98
Newsletter editing, 103,134

Nursing homes, volunteers, 28-29
　medical ministry, 3-6
　visiting, 11-12

Parents. *See* Family
Pasadena, California, 31-34,118
Pastors, 44
　hospital chaplaincy, 86-87
　interim, 95-98,138
　in New Zealand, 76-77,97-98
　in Santa Cruz, 52-53
　visitation and counseling, 76
　work in retirement, 52,95-98,107
　on Yavapai-Apache Indian Reservation, 71-72
Patience, 10
Peace Links, 16
Personal relationships. *See also* Family; Marriage
　helping friends, 23
　importance of, 60,141,164
　loneliness, 166
　in nursing homes, 29
　with young, 60
Peru, 105-106
Pets, 40,140
Philippines, 36
Planning, 1,50
　age of retirement, 148
　appreciation of life, 113
　deceleration of work, 58-59,60
　exercise and recreation, 60
　financial, 25
　holistic approach, 150
　importance of, 161
　mutability, 60
　relationships, 60
　spirituality, 50,84
　timing of retirement, 22
　volunteering in, 82,147-148
Political issues
　Bread for the World, 17
　fair housing laws, 72
　family and, 127-128
　immigration, 72

Political issues *(continued)*
Peace Links, 16
Prayer, 125
Prostitute rescue project, 40-41
Psalm 92:14, 2,37,144
Psalm 119:67, 71,138

Reading, 126-127
Real estate sales, 97
Recording books on tape, 28-29
Recreation. *See* Exercise and recreation; *specific activities*
Relationships. *See* Personal relationships
Religion. *See* Church; Spirituality
Relocation, 83,93,106,110,118-119
Remarriage, 50,55
Retirement
  health and, 93
  insights for productive, 161-166
  losses and gains, 59
  role models, 152
  statistics, 1
Retirement attitudes, 150
Retirement communities
  audiovisual program, 61-64
  volunteering in, 45,54,87,103
  Westminster Gardens, 18-19,27, 45,61-64,75-76,82,155-159
  Writers' Group, 155-159
Retirement planning. *See* Planning
Retirement support group, 44
Ritual of remembrance, 66-67
Role models, 152

Schools, volunteering in, 29
The Seventh Trouble (Gooding), 155
Shadow Hills, California, 96-97
Shadows from the Rising Sun (Lindholm), 37
Shingles, 125-126
Speer, Faye, 39-42

Spirituality, 24,25,80,84.
  See also Church
  aging and, 151
  baptism, 124
  caregiver for Alzheimer's spouse, 9-10
  grief and, 120-121
  health and, 144
  hospital chaplaincy, 88
  illness and, 126,133
  importance of, 164-165
  prayer, 125
  relationships and, 141
  retirement advice, 50
  ritual of remembrance, 66-67
Spouse. *See* Marriage
Stars in His Eyes (Gray), 53
Stereotypes, 150,151
Stewardship training, 35-38
Stomach cancer, 131-132
Suicide, 120
Support groups
  for grief, 93
  retirement, 44

Tajima, Ted, 131-135
Taylor, Marabelle, 3-6
Teaching, 154
  in Christian giving, 35-38
  English, 15-16
  English as a Second Language, 17, 101-102,135
  in Japan, 99-100,103-104
  literacy, 103
  planning for retirement, 57-59
  in retirement, 91,101-103
  tutoring children, 138-139
Telephone helpline, 16-17,49
Tennis, 73
Tentmaking ministries, 143,145
Thurman, Bob and Peggy, 147-152
Timothy 5:8, 9
Today's Tentmakers (Christy), 143
Tournier, Paul, 148

Travel, 18,48,49-50,78,87-88,92, 93,107-108,132-133
  Elderhostel, 13,23-24,119
  to visit family, 139-140
Tsuneishi, Arthur, 137
Tutoring children, 138-139
TV, closed-circuit, 61-64

University of Tennessee, 147-148

van Lierop, Peter, 1,2,85-89
Video network, in retirement communities, 61-64
Vietnamese, 138-139
Visitation, 76,149
  nursing homes, 11-12
Volunteering, 1-2. *See also* Community service
  American Association of University Women, 17
  book fair, 23-24
  Bread for the World, 17
  in church, 12-13,18,19,24,32-33, 41-42,43-44,92,111,119,145
    administration, 134-135
    editing newsletter, 134
    visitation and transportation, 82-84,149
    women's organizations, 124-125
  food banks, 41
  Habitat for Humanity, 34
  helping elderly, 49
  in hospitals, 23

Volunteering *(continued)*
  husband and wife as team, 151-152
  importance of, 161-162
  library work, 22-23
  in nursing homes, 28-29
    medical ministry, 3-6
    visiting, 11-12
  peace activism, 16
  in planning for retirement, 147-148
  prostitute rescue project, 40-41
  recording books on tapes, 28-29
  in retirement communities, 45,54, 87
  teaching, 18
    English, 15-16
    English as a Second Language classes, 17
    literacy, 103
    tutoring children, 138-139
  telephone helpline, 16-17,49

Walking, 12
Wedding anniversary, 78-79
Westminster Gardens, 18-19,27,45, 61-64,75-76,82,155-159
Wilson, Christy, Jr., 143-146
Women's emergency shelter, 18
Woodworking, 73
Worrying, 10
Writing, 53,143,144-145,155-159

Yavapai-Apache Indians, 71-73

Order Your Own Copy of
This Important Book for Your Personal Library!

ADVENTURES IN SENIOR LIVING
Learning How to Make Retirement Meaningful and Enjoyable

_____ in hardbound at $29.95 (ISBN: 0-7890-0253-1)

_____ in softbound at $14.95 (ISBN: 0-7890-0254-X)

COST OF BOOKS_____

OUTSIDE USA/CANADA/
MEXICO: ADD 20%_____

POSTAGE & HANDLING_____
(US: $3.00 for first book & $1.25
for each additional book)
Outside US: $4.75 for first book
& $1.75 for each additional book)

SUBTOTAL_____

IN CANADA: ADD 7% GST_____

STATE TAX_____
(NY, OH & MN residents, please
add appropriate local sales tax)

FINAL TOTAL_____
(If paying in Canadian funds,
convert using the current
exchange rate. UNESCO
coupons welcome.)

☐ **BILL ME LATER:** ($5 service charge will be added)
(Bill-me option is good on US/Canada/Mexico orders only;
not good to jobbers, wholesalers, or subscription agencies.)

☐ Check here if billing address is different from
shipping address and attach purchase order and
billing address information.

Signature_____

☐ **PAYMENT ENCLOSED: $**_____

☐ **PLEASE CHARGE TO MY CREDIT CARD.**

☐ Visa   ☐ MasterCard   ☐ AmEx   ☐ Discover
          ☐ Diner's Club

Account # _____

Exp. Date _____

Signature _____

Prices in US dollars and subject to change without notice.

NAME _____

INSTITUTION _____

ADDRESS _____

CITY _____

STATE/ZIP _____

COUNTRY _____ COUNTY (NY residents only) _____

TEL _____ FAX _____

E-MAIL_____
May we use your e-mail address for confirmations and other types of information? ☐ Yes   ☐ No

Order From Your Local Bookstore or Directly From
The Haworth Press, Inc.
10 Alice Street, Binghamton, New York 13904-1580 • USA
TELEPHONE: 1-800-HAWORTH (1-800-429-6784) / Outside US/Canada: (607) 722-5857
FAX: 1-800-895-0582 / Outside US/Canada: (607) 772-6362
E-mail: getinfo@haworth.com
PLEASE PHOTOCOPY THIS FORM FOR YOUR PERSONAL USE.

BOF96

NEW AND SOON-TO-BE PUBLISHED BOOKS FROM HAWORTH RELIGION, MINISTRY & PASTORAL CARE

TAKE 20% OFF EACH BOOK! *Special Sale!*

THE PASTORAL CARE OF DEPRESSION
A Guidebook
Binford W. Gilbert, PhD

Focuses on the people who become depressed and the skilled pastors who choose to treat depression. Pastors, pastoral counselors, chaplains, clergy, and psychiatrists and psychologists will learn more about the significant role religious confidantes can play in helping depressed people.

$29.95 hard. ISBN: 0-7890-0264-7.
$19.95 soft. ISBN: 0-7890-0265-5.
Available Winter 1997/98. Approx. 130 pp. with Index.

ADVENTURES IN SENIOR LIVING
Learning How to Make Retirement Meaningful and Enjoyable
Rev. J. Lawrence Driskill, STD

Helps you prepare for the opportunities, needs, problems, and challenges that retirement often brings. Retirees share with you a wide range of retirement ideas that pertain to volunteer work, travel, selecting your living arrangements, and getting involved in your community.

$29.95 hard. ISBN: 0-7890-0253-1.
$14.95 soft. ISBN: 0-7890-0254-X.
Available Winter 1997/98.
Approx. 190 pp. with Index.

WHEN LIFE MEETS DEATH
Stories of Death and Dying
Thomas William Shane, DDiv

This book 'tells the story' from the perspective of those who are immersed in the experience. Some are as common as the expected death of an elderly and ailing parent, while others are as traumatic as the loss of a loved one in the Oklahoma City bombing disaster. They are tales about the meaning and the mystery of people who must face the death of someone they love.

$39.95 hard. ISBN: 0-7890-0289-2.
$19.95 soft. ISBN: 0-7890-0290-6.
Available Winter 1997/98. Approx. 142 pp. with Index.

THE HEART OF PASTORAL COUNSELING
Healing Through Relationship, Revised Edition
Richard Dayringer, ThD

On the first edition:
"A comprehensive volume that offers concrete help and provides ladders for those suffering counseling pitfalls."
—Ministry

$39.95 hard. ISBN: 0-7890-0172-1
$19.95 soft. ISBN: 0-7890-0421-6.
Available Winter 1997/98. Approx. 209 pp. with Index.
Features 4 appendixes, charts/figures, diagnostic criteria, and a bibliography.

THE EIGHT MASKS OF MEN
A Practical Guide in Spiritual Growth for Men of the Christian Faith
Rev. Dr. Frederick G. Grosse

This book will encourage you to come out from behind your mask of solitude and loneliness—one of man's most obtrusive masks—and reach out for help and community.

$39.95 hard. ISBN: 0-7890-0415-1.
$16.95 soft. ISBN: 0-7890-0416-X.
Available Winter 1997/98. Approx. 181 pp. with Index.
Features anecdotal stories and excerpts by men who have undergone spiritual group work and an appendix of biblical references for spiritual growth.

VISA, MASTERCARD, DISCOVER, AMERICAN EXPRESS & DINERS CLUB WELCOME!

CALL OUR TOLL-FREE NUMBER: 1-800-HAWORTH
US & Canada only / 8am—5pm ET; Monday-Friday
Outside US/Canada: + 607-722-5857

FAX YOUR ORDER TO US: 1-800-895-0582
Outside US/Canada: + 607-771-0012

E-MAIL YOUR ORDER TO US: getinfo@haworth.com

VISIT OUR WEB SITE AT: www.haworth.com

The Haworth Press, Inc.
10 Alice Street,
Binghamton, New York 13904-1580 USA

AGING AND GOD
Spiritual Pathways to Mental Health in Midlife and Later Years
Harold G. Koenig, MD, MHSc

Over 500 Pages!

"The text is user-friendly.... Statistics are graphed or charted but also explained well."
—*Church & Synagogue Libraries*
$79.95 hard. ISBN: 1-56024-423-2.
$19.95 soft. ISBN: 1-56024-424-0. 1994. 544 pp. with Indexes.

HORRIFIC TRAUMATA
A Pastoral Response to the Post-Traumatic Stress Disorder
N. Duncan Sinclair, MDiv

"Outlines how pastoral counselors and others can help heal the isolation and trauma and promote growth."
—*Library Journal*
$39.95 hard. ISBN: 1-56024-293-0.
$12.95 soft. ISBN: 1-56024-294-9. 1993. 120 pp. with Index.

VICTIMS OF DEMENTIA
Services, Support, and Care
William Michael Clemmer, PhD

"Common sense approach, easy reading, specific day-to-day details of operation, and extensive appendixes."
—*Clinical Gerontologist*
$39.95 hard. ISBN: 1-56024-264-7.
$19.95 soft. ISBN: 1-56024-265-5. 1993. 155 pp. with Index.

RELIGION AND THE FAMILY
When God Helps
Edited by Laurel Arthur Burton, ThD

"Affords practical approaches to making faith an important part of therapy."
—*The American Journal of Family Therapy*
$39.95 hard. ISBN: 1-56024-192-6.
$19.95 soft. ISBN: 1-56024-197-7. 1992. 215 pp. with Index.

GROWING UP
Pastoral Nurture for the Later Years
Thomas B. Robb, ThD

"Gives the reader some searching insight into the personal and spiritual dimensions of growing up and growing old."
—*NAVAC*
$39.95 hard. ISBN: 1-56024-072-5.
$12.95 soft. ISBN: 1-56024-073-3. 1991. 148 pp. with Index.

CALL OUR TOLL-FREE NUMBER: 1-800-HAWORTH
US & Canada only / 8am-5pm ET; Monday-Friday
Outside US/Canada: + 607-722-5857

FAX YOUR ORDER TO US: 1-800-895-0582
Outside US/Canada: + 607-771-0012

E-MAIL YOUR ORDER TO US: getinfo@haworth.com

VISIT OUR WEB SITE AT: www.haworth.com

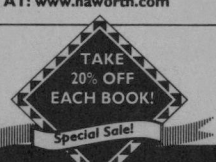

TAKE 20% OFF EACH BOOK! *Special Sale!*

Order Today and Save!

TITLE	ISBN	REGULAR PRICE	20%-OFF PRICE

- Discount good only in US, Canada, and Mexico and not good in conjunction with any other offer.
- Discount not good outside US, Canada, and Mexico.
- Individual orders outside US, Canada, and Mexico must be prepaid by check, credit card, or money order.
- Postage & handling: US: $3.00 for first book & $1.25 for each additional book; Outside US: $4.75 for first book & $1.75 for each additional book.

NAME _____

ADDRESS _____

_____

CITY _____

STATE _____ ZIP _____

COUNTRY _____

COUNTY (NY residents only) _____

TEL _____ FAX _____

E-MAIL _____
May we use your e-mail address for confirmations and other types of information? ( ) Yes ( ) No

- In Canada: Add 7% for GST before postage & handling.
- Outside USA, Canada, and Mexico: Add 20%
- MN, NY, and OH residents: Add appropriate local sales tax.
- If paying in Canadian funds, please use the current exchange rate to convert total to Canadian dollars.
- Payment in UNESCO coupons welcome.
- Please allow 3-4 weeks for delivery after publication.

❏ **BILL ME LATER** ($5 service charge will be added).
(Bill-me option available on US/Canadian/Mexican orders only. Not good for subscription agencies. Service charge is waived for booksellers/jobbers/wholesalers.)

Signature _____

❏ **PAYMENT ENCLOSED** _____
(Payment must be in US or Canadian dollars by check or money order drawn on a US or Canadian bank.)

❏ **PLEASE CHARGE TO MY CREDIT CARD:**
❏ VISA ❏ MASTERCARD ❏ AMEX ❏ DISCOVER ❏ DINERS CLUB

Account # _____ Exp Date _____

Signature _____

(10) 06/97 BBC97

The Haworth Press, Inc.
10 Alice Street, Binghamton, New York 13904-1580 USA